A POX ON THE PROVINCES

A POX ON THE PROVINCES

Proceedings of the 12th Congress of the British Society for the History of Medicine

Editors:
Roger Rolls
Jean & John R. Guy

Bath University Press

Designed by Bird Publications

Printed by Redwood Press Limited, Melksham, Wiltshire

Published by Bath University Press, Claverton Down, Bath

ISBN 0 86197 112 4

Contents

List of Contributors

John H. Cule, MA, MD, FRCGP. Lecturer in the History of Medicine, University of Wales College of Medicine.

Sir David Innes Williams, MD, MCh, FRCS. President of the Royal Society of Medicine.

Meyrick Emrys-Roberts, MB. B.Chir. Retired General Medical Practitioner

John R. Guy, BA, Ph.D, ARHistS. Archivist, Yeovil District Hospital

John Kirkup, BA, FRCS, DHMSA. Curator of the Instrument Collection, Royal College of Surgeons, London

Clive Charlton, MB, MS, FRCS. Consultant Urological Surgeon, Royal United Hospital, Bath

Jean Guy, MA, MB, B.Chir, DMRD, FFR, FRCR, DHMSA. Consultant Radiologist, Yeovil District Hospital

John Tricker, MB, BS, FRCS. Consultant Orthopaedic Surgeon, Yeovil District Hospital

Christine Hillam, BA, PhD. Hon. Research Fellow, Department of Dental Sciences, University of Liverpool

Nigel Lightfoot, MSc, MB, BS, MRCPath. Consultant Microbiologist, Newcastle-upon-Tyne Public Health Laboratory

James Skeggs, Accessions Officer, Somerset Record Office, Taunton

Audrey Heywood, MB, ChB, Research Registrar, Department of Renal Medicine, Southmead Hospital, Bristol

Roger Rolls, MA, MB, B.Chir. General Medical Practitioner, Bath

Joan Lane, MA, PhD, FSA. Senior Research Fellow, Centre for the Study of Social History, University of Warwick

Peter Wallis, PhD. Director of the Project for Historical Biobibliography (PHIBB) Newcastle-upon-Tyne

Sholem Glaser, FRCS. Retired Consultant Urological Surgeon, Royal United Hospital, Bath

John B. Lyons, MD (NUI), FRCPI. Professor of the History of Medicine, Royal College of Surgeons in Ireland

Terence Turner, OBE, M.Pharm, FRPS, FLS, MCPP Senior Lecturer, Welsh School of Pharmacy, University of Wales, Cardiff

Anne Young, BSc, MB, BS, DPM, DHMSA. Retired Psychiatrist

Hugh Torrens, BA, PhD. Lecturer in the Centre for the History of Science and Technology, University of Keele

Patricia Maureen Craig, BA, MB. Course Tutor, The Open University

Owen Dudley Edwards, BA, FRHistS. Reader in History, University of Edinburgh

INTRODUCTION & ACKNOWLEDGEMENTS

Until comparatively recently, scant attention was paid to the history and evolution of English provincial medicine. With one or two exceptions, this collection of essays, first presented at the 12th Congress of the British Society for the History of Medicine held at Bath University in April 1988, is strongly biased towards the practice of medicine in the provinces, chronologically commencing with John Cule's paper on Romano-Druidic medicine and ending with Owen Dudley Edwards' commentary on the provincial doctor as exemplified in the works of Arthur Conan Doyle.

A particularly provincial feature of our medical heritage, the cottage hospital, is the focus of a study by Meyrick Emrys-Roberts who considers the contenders for the earliest of these institutions. David Innes Williams' review of the rise of specialist medicine demonstrates the influence of provincial practitioners and related institutions beyond the confines of the metropolis. Four other papers deal with individual specialities. The rise of the dental profession is a particularly provincial phenomenon originating, as Christine Hillam shows, from diverse sources. Clive Charlton's study of the development of the flexible urethral catheter suggests that this indispensible device owes as much to improvements in the technology of rubber manufacture as it does to the ingenuity of individual urologists. Jean Guy looks at the emerging speciality of radiology in two West of England hospitals and in particular the conflicts and misunderstandings which arose between the early radiologists and their clinical colleagues. The application of X-rays revolutionised the management of bone injury but John Tricker's paper on the history of fracture treatment shows a remarkably sophisticated level of management being practised long before Röntgen's discovery in 1895. Fractures were amongst the injuries treated at the Bath Casualty Hospital founded in 1788. This little known institution, the subject of the paper by John Kirkup, is probably the earliest example of a specialist accident hospital in Great Britain.

Another type of medical institution particularly associated with rural settings, the isolation hospital, has departed relatively recently from the milieu of medicine and is still remembered by many of the older generation with a degree of dread and loathing, as John Guy reminds us in his study, "The Shadow of the Fever Van." In earlier times, contagious fevers were most often associated with the term 'plague'. Nigel Lightfoot and James Skeggs have examined a number of sixteenth and seventeenth century Somerset parish records. Their paper highlights the dangers of interpreting the term 'plague' too literally. A similar problem of interpretation presented itself to Audrey Heywood in her attempt to indentify cases of lead poisoning admitted to the Bath General Hospital during the eighteenth century. In general, her task was made easier by the availability of extant case descriptions, but the problem of semiotic ambiguity remains. Her experimental work into the possible mode of action of spa therapy provides an intriguing explanation of Bath's reputation for successfully curing certain types of disorder during its heyday as a health resort. Roger Rolls briefly surveys the hydro-therapeutic techniques which evolved at Bath and which provide an example of the importance of spa towns in the popularisation of physical methods of treatment.

Historical studies of Bath have hitherto tended to focus primarily on its role as a place of diversion and frivolity for fashionable eighteenth century society, ignoring its attraction to a scientific community which became active there in the latter eighteenth and early nineteenth centuries. Hugh Torrens' study of the establishment of three vigorous philosophical societies at Bath, each of which was supported by a considerable membership of medical men, would seem to suggest that the city was not the scientific wilderness that some historians have hitherto suggested.

A scientific education as we know it today did not exist in the eighteenth century where university courses were still firmly grounded in the classics. Their classical educational background may explain why so many provincial physicians distinguished themselves in cultural activities which had little or no relationship to their job as doctors. Such diversity of interest and talent shows itself in the lives of two eighteenth century physicians described respectively by Sholem Glaser and Jack Lyons. Glaser's study reveals Dr Henry Harington's interest and ability as a musician while Lyons' examination of the King's professor of medicine in Dublin University, Dr Edward Hill, focusses on the physician's preoccupation with the literary works of John Milton.

Many rural areas were relatively isolated from orthodox medical practitioners and frequently had to provide for themselves. Self medication was popular in an age which antedated medical insurance and the National Health Service. Terry Turner's paper, "Secret Nostrums", which examines the cult of the proprietary medicine and Anne Young's survey of domestic medicine chests (so often mislabelled as apothecaries' cabinets by antique dealers) provide two contrasting studies in home doctoring.

The lack of any comprehensive national register of eighteenth century medical practitioners has prompted several medical historians to attempt to compile such a work of reference. This has finally come to fruition with the appearance of the PHIBB database of 18th Century Medics, now available in print and in its second edition. Its compiler, Peter Wallis, gives here an outline of its development and format. Much of the information has come from apprenticeship records. Apprenticeships formed the backbone of medical education for the bulk of British doctors before the Medical Acts of the mid-nineteenth century and Joan Lane's paper provides a comprehensive appraisal of the system during the eighteenth century. The demise of medical apprenticeship was one of a number of changes in the nineteenth century affecting the status of the medical profession. Pat Craig examines the press coverage of three BMA meetings held at Bristol in the early and later years of the nineteenth century and notes a considerable difference of emphasis reflecting a changing perception of the doctor's role. How that role was perceived, at least by one well-known practitioner, is explored by Owen Dudley Edwards in his fascinating contribution.

A successful Congress is more than a series of papers well delivered by lecturers who keep to time. The Bath Medical History Group which was invited to organise the 12th Congress of the British Society for the History of Medicine is small in numbers (less than thirty) and with a widely scattered membership (from Wantage to Penzance). That the Congress was generally acclaimed a success is due in no small measure to the enthusiasm and hard work of all the members of that Group who willingly contributed their time and talents. In particular we wish to acknowledge the help of Nigel Naunton Davies, the Congress Treasurer, also Bruno Bubna Kasteliz, Myles McNulty, Clive Quinnell, Jeffrey Morgan, Meyrick Emrys-Roberts and Kevin Craig, who chaired the six sessions of the academic programme, along with Ben Davis and John Kirkup, who presided over the plenary sessions with which the Congress began and closed.

We are particularly grateful to both the American Museum at Claverton Manor, and especially the University of Bath, for the facilities they provided. In particular, we thank the School of Pharmacy and Pharmacology, Jackie Cressey, the University's Conference Officer, and Margaret Hansen, whose dual role as member of the Group and a lecturer in the School of Pharmacy proved invaluable. We also wish to acknowledge the generosity of Syntex and Glaxo Laboratories, Ltd. for their great help in mounting the Congress, and the assistance of Dr P.M. Pollak, the Revd Francis Buxton, and the Gentlemen's Catch Club.

Readers of this volume who were present at the Congress will notice a few changes from the original list of contributions. The paper "Evidence for Injuries and Arthritis in Skeletal Populations", read by Juliet Rogers, was not submitted to the editors for inclusion. John Cule's paper "The Revd John Wesley and Alternative Medicine" had been promised to another publication, but Dr Cule kindly offered a substitute with which this volume opens. We also include two papers, by Meyrick Emrys-Roberts and Sholem Glaser, which were prepared for the Congress but in the event not delivered. The publication of these Proceedings has been undertaken by the University of Bath Press and we are particularly grateful for the help and assistance of John Lamble and Bob Bragg in the preparation of the volume.

There is not one way of thinking and writing about a subject as vast and inexhaustible as the history of medicine. The biennial British Congresses provide an opportunity to explore a variety of its aspects in some depth. Bath seemed a natural place in which to examine the subject of provincial medicine. We hope you will enjoy reading about it as much as the participants enjoyed the Congress.

Roger Rolls
Jean and John R. Guy

Editors

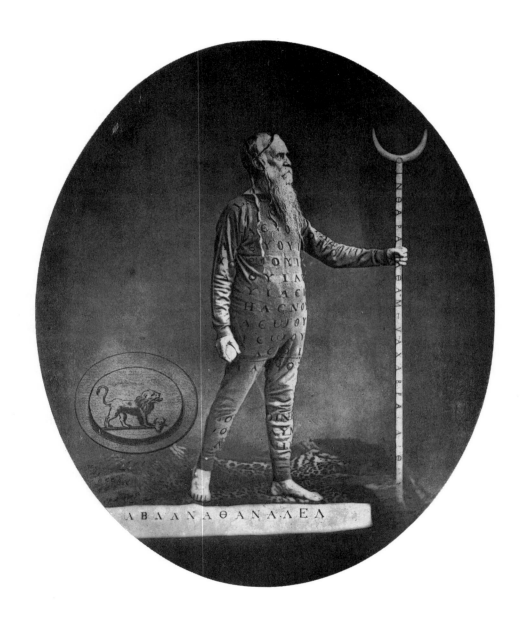

1. William Price, MRCS, LSA (1800 - 1893). Wearing the costume he believed was that of the ancient Welsh druids.

THE PROVINCE OF BRITAIN: Wales, druidic magic and Roman medicine

John Cule

It is perhaps a little surprising to find the druids described as "the most advanced of all intellectual classes among the peoples of ancient Europe beyond the Greek and Roman world".[1] The time of their ascendancy in Wales was about the second century BC. Their study is not helped by their having committed nothing of their learning to writing, although Caesar states that they were supposed to have used Greek lettering for other matters.[2] There is no evidence that their medical thinking was influenced by the Greeks, even though it has been suggested that they held similar opinions to those of the Pythagorean school on the transmigration of souls. The oral tradition for the transmission of knowledge, which has parallels amongst other ancient peoples, was not likely to survive unscathed in aural memory. We therefore have to rely for our information on their study of the nature of things, *natura rerum*, from alien Greek and Roman sources. These are sufficient to indicate that it was not only in the teaching of crafts that there was an oral tradition. Amongst a great deal of literature, written by others about the druids and much of it since their time, a composite but incomplete picture of their activities may be derived.[3]

Professor Tierney believes that the medico-magical side of the druids, so prominent in Pliny's *Natural History*, is the true historical basis of their influence and power.[4] Caius Plinius Secundus, Pliny the Elder, was born in Como about 23 AD and died in 79 AD. He completed the text of his *Natural History* by 77 AD and the oldest copy known is that of the eighth or ninth century. Little has been discovered of Pliny's sources although Divitiacus, the Gaulish druidic friend of Caesar and Cicero has been suggested as an informant, acting perhaps indirectly through an intermediary such as Cicero. Chadwick, however, thinks this is unlikely and she also does not regard Posidonius, whose writings Cicero made use of in his books, as the probable source of the medico-magical lore with which Pliny credits the druids.[5] Although Polyhistor and Timaeus are quoted by Pliny elsewhere, neither of these seem to have provided any contributions of a medical nature. Even with such doubts that the uncertainties of his sources bring, it is on Pliny that we have to rely for what medical information there is in relation to druidic practice.

Pliny does give some account of the druids in relation to their magical and medical practices, subjects to which he devoted much of his writing. In describing these druidic practices he was therefore but illustrating his general interest. As early as the second century BC the druids had a reputation outside Gaul, suggesting an antiquity of possibly a century or more. By Caesar's time they were "an organised and powerful body having important educational, judicial, political, as well as religious functions; moreover the order included various kinds of officials, priests, prophets and poets, while we gather that some of its members were free to devote themselves entirely to the duties of government and international affairs"[6] Caesar, Strabo and Diodorus Siculus, writing in the first century BC owe their information to Posidonius and no mention is made by them of any medical or even magico-medical function. The philosophical activity is mentioned by Cicero, writing of the druids in Gaul.

> "I myself knew one of them, Divitiacus, the Aeduan, your guest and eulogist, who declared that he was acquainted with the system of nature, which the Greeks call natural philosophy *(physiologia)*."

And Caesar, himself, includes Britain in the sphere of druidism.

> "It is believed that their rule of life was discovered in Britain and transferred thence to Gaul; and those today who would study the subject more accurately journey, as a rule, to Britain to learn it."[8]

Tacitus' well-known passage which describes the terrorising of the Roman soldiery by the British druids of Anglesey, during the raid on that island by Suetonius Paulinus in 60 AD does not mention them in the biography of his father-in-law Agricola, who administered Britain for seven years from 78 AD, although this work was written before *The Annals*.[9] Paulinus in wiping up a focus of material resistance was also "wiping out a native cult of which the influence was much more pervasive than any ancient author hints."[10]

Pliny, who is the only author to have stressed their medical skills - an art he generally admired - records our debt to the Romans for having put an end to "the monstrous cult" proscribed by a decree of the Emperor Tiberius against "their druids and the whole tribe of diviners and physicians."[11] His descriptions of the medico-magical practices of the druids are to be found in Books XVI and XXIV of his *Natural History*. In them is described the ritual necessary for the collection of mistletoe by the druids and its use "taken in drink" to impart "fecundity to barren animals" and "as an antidote for all poisons".[12] The mistletoe was to be gathered...

> "with due religious ceremony, if possible on the sixth day of the moon ... They call the mistletoe by a name meaning, in their language, the all-healing. Having made preparation for sacrifice and a banquet beneath the trees, they bring thither two white bulls, whose horns are bound then for the first time. Clad in a white robe, the priest ascends the tree and cuts the mistletoe with a golden sickle, and it is received by others in a white cloak. Then they kill the victims, praying that God will render this gift of his propitious to those whom he has granted it."[13]

Pliny's references to mistletoe *(viscum)* as *omnia sanantem appellantes suo vocabulo* has suggested to some an association with the Welsh word *holliach*, meaining literally "perfectly well" or "all healthy" and which is also translated by Bodwyn Anwyl as mistletoe. There are examples in Welsh literature of *holliach* having the same meaning as the English "tutsan".[14] *The Shorter Oxford English Dictionary* gives "tutsan" as a late Middle English name applied to plants on account of their healing virtue. It formerly applied to *Agnus castus* (the Chaste Tree or Abraham's Balm) and now to *Hypericum androseum*, or the Shrubby Saint John's Wort. In its formalised version, "Three sprigs of the herb 'all-heal' proper", it is today used as the crest of the Royal Society of Medicine.

There were also instructions for the collection of *selago*, the smoke of which was said to be good for diseases of the eye. The *selago* is said to be similar to savin, *Juniperus sabina*.[15] This had to be gathered "without the use of iron and by passing the right hand through the left sleeve of the tunic, as though in the act of committing a theft. The clothing must be white, the feet washed and bare, and an offering of wine and bread made before the gathering."[16]

The marsh plant, *samolus*, to be gathered "with the left hand, when fasting", was used as a charm against diseases of cattle. Its gatherer was enjoined not to look behind him, nor to lay the plant anywhere other than in the drinking troughs.[17] Hugh Davies gives the following description of *samolus*.

> Samolus; Brookweed; *Claerlys*.
> *S Valerandi*; Brookweed, Water Pimpernel; *Claerlys*,
> *Sammwl, Samylen*. In marshes and near springs.[18]

With the Roman legions there came to Wales a new approach to medicine. By the middle of the first century AD, the Welsh were being contained in their native hills by the XXth Legion at *Glevum*, the Severn crossing at Gloucester and by the XIVth Legion at *Viroconium*, the Severn crossing at Wroxeter. About 80 AD, Julius Frontinus sent the Second Legion to Caerleon. A network of forts spread through Wales. There was a walled town at Caerwent, about eight miles east of the Second Legion Fortress at Caerleon on Usk. Carmarthen *(Moridunum)* in the extreme west was also walled, and began its development as a cantonal capital about 130 AD.

About 75 AD the new capital for the Silures, *Venta Silurum*, was founded at Caerwent as part of the policy of Romanisation of the native population. It reached its greatest prosperity during the second century, to decline in common with other British Roman towns during the fourth. In its prime it was protected by the large fortress at Caerleon, which lost its importance when, in the third century, the old fortress at Cardiff was rebuilt as a coastal protection against seaborne raiders. The Romans in their fortresses and in the town of Caerwent have left archaeological evidence of their interest in medicine and hygiene.

There are references throughout classical literature that reveal a high standard of achievement in the preservation of health and in the Roman care for the sick and wounded. It has been said that the Romans left only three valuable permanent legacies in Britain; the traditional site of London, the Roman roads and Celtic Christianity.[19] They certainly brought with them many more things of great value, even if much of it did not rub off on the natives. Amongst these was a standard of medicine and public health new to Britain.

A description of the Graeco-Roman medical and surgical instruments, with special reference to those found in Wales has been written by Peter Thomas.[20] The finds have been mainly of different varieties of probes, spatulae *(ligulae)*, spoons, tweezers and forceps; in particular a bronze uvula forceps *(staphylagra)* from Caerwent and a sharp hook *(haemulus acutus)*, a bronze shears and a chatelaine at Shrewsbury. For medical and pharmaceutical use there are examples of a small folding balance *(libra)* and a bronze steelyard *(statera)* also at Shrewsbury.

The tradition of medical care was nurtured by a long succession of emperors. It was said that Alexander Severus (222-235 AD) cared more for his soldiers than for himself. He recognised that this reputation at least paid dividends in upholding the fighting man's morale, the support of which was neglected at the commander's peril.

Richmond describes the military structure in the first and second centuries as consisting of "the legions, composed of Roman citizens and each forming a battalion some 5,500 strong; and the auxiliary regiments, raised in the outer provinces and organised as cavalry, infantry or part-mounted units, each containing in round figures a thousand or five hundred men. Later there came in addition irregular formations of cavalry and infantry, ... but it remains uncertain how the medical services for these were organised."[21]

As the Roman occupation of Britain was consolidated, conscription and recruitment to the Roman army took place from amongst the native inhabitants. This was in accordance with

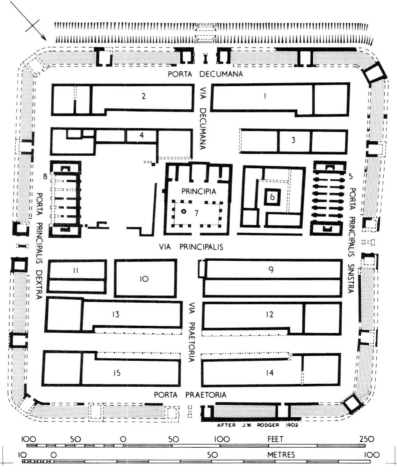

2. The Roman Fort at Gelligaer in Glamorgan. The building marked 4 on the plan is believed to have been the Valetudinarium. *(Crown Copyright Royal Commission on Ancient and Historical Monuments for Wales)*

the general policy of the empire. During the second century, besides the legions, there were many auxilliary regiments in Britain. British regiments were recruited and took part in Trajan's campaigns. "Men from Wales and northern Britain could be sent to the Danubian provinces" to help police the new territories that were being added.[22]

Hospitals were an important part of the system. The *valetudinaria* of several legionary fortresses have been excavated and conform to a broadly similar general plan. There is a good example in Wales at Caerleon. The limited excavation at Caerleon revealed the small wards on the outer side of the peripheral corridor that enclosed the central square and these were probably grouped in threes, whilst on the inner side they were in pairs, with vestibules between each section. The plan followed that of the original tented hospital, the sixty tents or wards relating to the sixty *centuriae* into which the legion was divided. Ten patients per ward suggested an expected 10% casualty list.[21] However, Caerleon itself was so far behind any fighting front that it was unlikely to have dealt with anything other than the routine sick. No latrines were found, but a small section of drain indicates that - as usual - there were such sanitary arrangements. Only one small room was found to have been heated, and that not until the middle of the second century AD. A timber framed hospital had already been on the site from 75-80 AD until the beginning of the second century, when the hospital was rebuilt in stone. Repairs including re-roofing and re-flooring were carried out at intervals during its occupation until the buildings were systematically dismantled in the last years of the third century.[23]

There appears to have been a small hospital at Usk *(Burrium)*. Another at Pen Llystyn, consisted of "a simple range of ten rooms opening on to a veranda with another room at one end extending over the veranda."[24] It is possible that a building at the smaller military fort in Gelligaer could have been a *valetudinarium*.[25] An auxiliary fort with accommodation for a *cohors quingenaria* of 480 infantry would have warranted it. The bath buildings at Gelligaer are identifiable. The custom was to induce the bather to sweat by a form of heating similar to that of a Turkish bath, scrape off the sweat with scrapers *(strigiles)* and apply ointments. The rooms were carefully graded in temperature. There were hot and cold baths and dressing rooms. The floors were heated by underground hypocausts, connected to a furnace, and there was a piped water supply. The ceremonial of the bath, a place as well for other relaxations such as gambling, was under the patronage of Fortuna, to whom there is a dedication in one of the legionary bath buildings at Caerleon.[25] No hospital is identifiable in the small fort at Caerhun, for which a good plan exists. It is more probable that one might be found at Caernarfon which, like Pen Llystyn, was large enough to hold a military cohort.

Whereas the Romans took great care to leave native customs and practices undisturbed, as long as they did not interfere with government, many Britons voluntarily adopted Roman ways. In the settled parts of Britain, land owners copied Roman villas within a generation of the conquest. Later on bath houses were added, a feature which had not been so readily accepted at first. As the towns grew, British craftsmen and traders joined the Roman inhabitants. It is now known that this process reached Carmarthen *(Moridunum)* the walling of which required permission from and direct communication with Rome. Roman citizenship continued to be extended until in 212 AD the privilege was given to all free-born provincials.

It is not known how widely held amongst the Romans abroad were the views that Celsus expressed on medicine. But it would seem likely that they are as representative as were his views on surgery, for which there is corroboration in the instruments and organisation of the Roman surgeon in the field. At the end of the *Prooemium*, Celsus writes that he is "of the opinion that the Art of Medicine ought to be rational, but to draw instruction from evident causes, all obscure ones being rejected from the practice of the Art, although not from the practitioner's study". This "useful" knowledge, which had been applied with typical Roman thoroughness and organisation to the provision of a military surgical service was surely equally acceptable in Roman medicine. There are some ideas of sympathetic magic, with such remedies as worms boiled in oil for the treatment of maggots in the ear, but unlike Pliny he does not give these prominence. Pliny claimed to prefer herbal simples but his medical books contain much simple magic used in the form of ritual during the exhibition of formulae containing animal as well as plant remedies. Superstition, which Pliny claims to scorn, permeates his collection of therapeutic records. Celsus's medicine is practical rather than speculative, of the body rather than the spirit.[26]

But, practical as the Roman military medicine was, religion still played a part in healing as it did for many of their subjects. On the right bank of the River Severn at Lydney, near the beginning of the Severn Bore, lie the ruins of a temple, erected in the late fourth century in honour of Nodens, a god of hunting and water; the equivalent of Nuadu of the Irish and Llud Llaw Eraint of the Welsh.[27] The name Nodens is conserved in "Nudd" of Gwyn ap Nudd, King of Annwn.[28] Alongside the temple court is an open fronted building divided into cells reminiscent of the type of structure where the sick slept whilst awaiting the healing dreams of cults such as that of Asclepius, which itself reached "a new magnificence during the second century". Nearby there are baths and a guest house. The names of the gods seem of common tradition and it is possible that the Greek cult of Asclepius, later adopted by the Romans, flourished at Lydney. Sick people went to such places to await in sleep the experience of communion with the god and his healing power. The practice was known as incubation. The purpose of the priestly guardians of the temple seems to have been in the nature of selection of the patient, the dying being rigorously excluded. The process invoked was in the dreams of specific cures by the god, who was traditionally attended by snakes. Another temple at Caerwent *(Venta Silurum)* is dedicated to Mars Ocelus Vellaunus, who might be related to the Mars Lenus of the Moselle, more famous for his healing than for war.[29] Sometimes the great god Mars himself was invoked for protection against severe pestilences. In such sacred places recourse could be had to the old religious methods by its devotees, or by those for whom the practical medicine of the army had failed.

An altar from Chester is dedicated in Greek to the "mighty saviour gods" by Hermogenes, believed to have been either a *medicus* in the XXth Legion or the personal physician of one of its senior officers.[30] There is another second century tablet, which was found nearby, on which a Dr Antiochus honours Asclepius, Hygeia and Panakeia.[31] The gods played important parts in Roman and in Celtic life.

The only Welsh doctor of this time for whom we have individual evidence is of the late fifth to the early sixth century. His death is commemorated by a tombstone inscription now in the parish churchyard of Llangian in Llyn.[32]

It is written vertically in three lines.[33]

MELI MEDICI
FILI MARTINI
I(A)CET

Professor I Ll.Foster regarded it as "possibly unique in Britain in its record of *medicus*".[34] This inscription, made in a manner alien to the orthodox Christianity of the period, is reminiscent in its filial form "N son of M lies here", of that of the Celtic tribal society. "N son of M" is a translation of the Irish formula, often carved in the fourth century Ogam script, which was particularly suited by its style for use on funerary monuments. Indeed, it did not need to be put to other literary use for the dominant Celtic tradition of the time was still oral and not written. Such Welsh memorials are distinguished from those of the continent by the name of the deceased appearing in the genitive case, ("the stone" being understood). The inscriptions followed the vertical line of the Ogam epitaph, even when Roman lettering was used. Even *hic iacet* was frequently written vertically and not horizontally. Often no burials can be found near these stones, indicating that they have been moved from their original sites to the protection of the churchyard.[35]

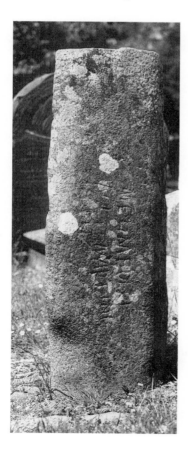

3. The Melus Stone in Llangian Churchyard, Gwynedd. Late 6th century. *(Crown Copyright Royal Commission on Ancient and Historical Monuments for Wales)*

Another stone has been reported from Lethnot, Angus, Tayside discovered originally during repairs to the church floors in the 1880's , which might refer to a *medicus*. The text is incomplete but the decipherable part reads:

FILII

MEDICII

This could be translated as either "the son of Medicius" or "the son of the doctor". If the word *medicus* was intended, the double I of the inscription is presumably in error.[36]

The tombstone of Melus is quite distinct from that of the *medicus ordinarius* of the Tungrian cohort in Britain found near Housesteads and now in Newcastle Museum. It does record another *medicus*, but in the continental style.

```
D.M

ANICIO

INCENVO

MEDICO

ORD.COH

I.TVNGR

VIX.AN.XXV.
```

This abbreviated inscription may be expanded and then translated thus.

D (is) M(anibus)
Anicio
Ingenuo
Medico
Ord(inario) Coh(ortis)
Primae Tungr(orum)
Vix(it) An(nis) XXV

To the gods of the Shades. Cinicius Ingenuus *medicus ordinarius* of the First Tungrian Cohort. He lived 25 years.[37]

The age of Melus *medicus*, the son of Martin was not recorded. He is still the first named medical practitioner in Wales, and his tombstone brings a solid primary source, writ in stone, to introduce its recorded medical history.

REFERENCES

1. Chadwick, N.K. *The Druids*, Cardiff, 1966, Preface p vii

2. Chadwick, op cit, p 42

3. Momigliano, Arnaldo, *Alien Wisdom*, Cambridge: Cambridge University Press, 1975, p 70; Piggott, S. *Ancient Europe*, Edinburgh: Edinburgh University Press, 1965, pp 226, 227, 230; See also Kendrick T.D. *The Druids*, London: Methuen & Co, 1927

4. Tierney, J.J. *Proceedings of the Royal Irish Academy*, **60**, Section C, No 5, Dublin, 1960, p 215

5. Chadwick, op cit, p 33

6. Kendrick T.D. *The Druids*, London: Methuen & Co, 1927, pp 98-99

7. Cicero, *De Divinatione*, I, XLI, 90 (Kendrick, p 80, from Judge Falconer's version, *Loeb Library*, London:1922)

8. Caesar, J. *De Bello Gallico*, VI, 13 (Kendrick, p 77, from H.J. Edwards' version, *Loeb Library*, 1917)

9. Tacitus, *Annals*, XIV, 30 (Kendrick, p 92, from translation by Church and Brodribb, London: 1876)

10. Richmond, I.A. *Roman Britain*, Penguin Books, Harmondsworth: (Pelican History of England 1), 1963, p 28

11. Pliny, *Naturalis Historia*, XXX, 13 (Kendrick, p 90)

12. ibid, XVI, 251 (Kendrick, pp 88/89)

13. ibid, XVI, 250-1 (Kendrick, p 89)
    (Loeb *tr* says they call the moon "all-healing")

14. Personal communication. The late Mr R. J. Thomas, editor, *Geiriadur Prifysgol Cymru*, 15th June, 1966

15. Dorland, W.A.N. *The American Illustrated Medical Dictionary*, 1938, Philadelphia and London, 18th ed

16. Pliny, *Nat Hist*, op cit, XXIV, 103 (Kendrick, p 89)

17. ibid, XXIV, 104 (Kendrick, p 89)

18. Davies, H. *Welsh Botanology*, London, 1813, p 24

19. Trevelyan, G.M. *History of England*, London, 1928, p 14

20. Thomas, P. *The Journal of the College of General Practitioners*, 1963, **6**, pp 495-502

21. Richmond, I.A. *Univ Durham Med Gaz*, June 1952, **46**, pp 2-6

22.   Simpson, G. *Britons and the Roman Army*, London, 1964, pp 116-7

23.   Threipland, L. Murray, *Arch Camb*, 1969
Boon, G.C. *Isca, The Roman Legionary Fortress at Caerleon Mon*, Cardiff: National Museum of Wales, 1972, pp 75-77

24.   Webster,G. *Roman Imperial Army*, London: Gregg Press 1969, p 217. Plan of Pen Llystyn on p 212, Fig 48

25.   Nash-Williams, V.E. *The Roman Frontier in Wales*, Cardiff, 1954, pp 133-137

26.   Spencer, W.G. *Celsus de Medicina*, Loeb Classical Library, 1961, p 41
Jones, W.H.S. *Pliny Natural History*, Loeb Classical Library, Vol 8, 1963

27.   Rees, A. & B. *Celtic Heritage*, London, 1961, pp 46 & 51

28.   Jones, T.G. *Welsh Folklore and Custom*, London, 1930, p 52

29.   Lane Fox, Robin, *Pagans and Christians*, Harmondsworth: Viking, 1986, pp 51-2 (also available in Penguin). He refers to 'special "incubatory" chambers at Lydney in Kent' (sic) ... 'where dreams were courted deliberately'. He must mean Lydney, Glos.
Richmond, I.A. *Roman Imperial Army*, op cit, pp 139-142. 192

30.   Webster, G. *Roman Imperial Army*, op cit, p 251, fn 6

31.   Nutton, Vivian. "A Greek Doctor at Chester" in *Journal of the Chester Archaeological Society*, **55**, 1968, pp 7-13. I am indebted to Dr Nutton for several references and his comment that these medical memorials suggest the possibility of a Roman hospital at Chester, possibly under the Cathedral. This paper also discusses the position of the *medicus ordinarius* in the Roman Army. See also Nutton, V. "Medicine and the Roman Army", *Medical History*, **13**, No 3, July 1969, pp 260-270

32.   Nash-Williams, V.E. *The Early Christian Monuments of Wales*, Cardiff, 1950. Caerns 92. Cited by Foster, I. Ll., & Daniel, Glyn, (eds) *Prehistoric and Early Wales*, London: Routledge & Kegan Paul, 1935, p 217

33.   Personal Communication. Rev A.O.J. Thomas, M.A. 23 Aug 1966

34.   Foster, I. Ll., & Daniel, Glyn, *Prehistoric & Early Wales*, op cit, p 217

35.   Alcock, L. "Wales in the fifth to seventh centuries", in Foster and Daniel, *Prehistoric & Early Wales*, pp 204-6

36.   *Cambridge Mediaeval Celtic Studies*, **9**, Summer, 1985, p 53

37.   Comrie, J.D. *History of Scottish Medicine*, London: 1932, Vol I, illust opp p 37

SPECIALISTS AND SPECIAL HOSPITALS

David Innes Williams

Increasing specialisation has been a dominant factor in medical practice throughout the past one hundred years, rapidly accelerating during the last twenty-five. The trend has frequently been decried and to it, along with high technology, has been attributed the decay of caring medicine. Yet its progress has been inexorable and through it major advances in treatment have been achieved. Specialist hospitals have been a feature of all our major cities, some founded in the eighteenth but mostly in the mid and late nineteenth century when they became absurdly numerous. Some were ephemeral but new foundations continued to attract charitable support up to the start of the National Health Service while special provision was made by local authorities for fevers and mental disorders from the very early period.

Both World Wars stimulated the establishment of specialist hospitals for care of the wounded. Many have now closed or merged with general hospitals as a result of professional or financial pressure but a few survive to preserve their lively tradition. This paper examines the relationship between the development of the special hospitals and the emergence of a recognised medical or surgical specialty. It is a very large subject of which I can only now give you a flavour. Indeed it is an area which requires a deeper study than I have yet been able to devote to it although my personal career had been closely bound up with specialist hospitals and with a maturing speciality.

The clinical specialists with which I am concerned are loosely coherent groups of doctors perceiving themselves as providing on a whole or part-time basis a clinical service distinct from the generality of medical care. The existence of a speciality is recognised by specialist associations and publications; the specialists themselves are identified by their hospital, university or institutional appointments, although almost all will in the earlier stages be involved in general medical, surgical or family practice as well.

It is of course axiomatic that a speciality can only exist where there is a sufficient body of relevant patients and sufficient funds from individual fees or public sources to support the specialist doctors. Financial factors, both positive and negative, have been important in the genesis and in the demise of specialities; they impinge upon the income of the doctor and on the charitably provided support of his hospital or dispensary but it would be a mistake to interpret the role of the doctors as dominated solely by the need to make money. Doctors have always liked to treat patients and more than can easily be found in private practice. They enjoy the exercise of their skill. Benefactors too may well have mixed motives and think of the public esteem which they may gain by their contributions but there is no reason to suppose that those who gave their money and time to the foundation of special hospitals were either more or less altruistic than the donors and fund raisers for the small charities of today. The doctor likes to think he has a special skill to offer, the benefactor likes a comprehensible objective in which his personal contribution would be identifiable.

Specialties can arise in a variety of ways, but there are certain common evolutionary patterns. In the first phase there are individual experts who, developing a particular interest, have narrowed their field of endeavour after a wider experience. Some attain considerable prominence and perhaps a Court Appointment. The qualities which Royalty looks for in its medical advisers are by no means always those which attract the esteem of their colleagues but at this stage, although there may be envy, there is no perception of a threat from a specialist development. The success of the individuals however stimulates the younger men to embark on a special field early in their careers seeking an opportunity to make their mark soon after completing their training, though often with the intention once they are established of practising more widely in medicine or surgery.

Surgical specialties have in general emerged earlier than medical since they have been associated with the acquisition of a particular skill or the invention of a new instrument. Surgeons were more actively entrepreneurial than the physicians and medical specialties more likely to follow the segregation of particular groups of patients on charitable or social grounds. In recent years however the technical skill now required by a physician in several fields as for instance catheterisation in cardiology or dialysis in nephrology is encouraging the growth of medical specialties, though at a time when it is too late to found a special hospital.

The emerging speciality soon becomes a recognised one when the pioneers pass on their skills to their pupils and assistants, but at the same time it becomes a threat to be resisted by the generalists. Hostility towards an interloper is perhaps a natural reaction though the strength of that reaction was, and often still is, surprising to those involved. The established general surgeon sees the speciality not simply as encouraging a contender for his practice but as questioning his competence, a slur on his reputation and an affront to his dignity. Thus we find from the 1830's onwards that the small band of physicians and surgeons of the general infirmaries, having achieved social prestige as well as practice from their appointments, resisted any dilution of their privilege by numerous recruits or by a motley crowd of specialists whom they castigated with extraordinary vituperation. Such people were branded as quacks, the ultimate wounding stigma.

Nevertheless, with a rapidly growing population, an expanding potential for medical and surgical treatment and a numerous body of young doctors, the trend to specialism was irresistible, even though for very many years the specialists were assigned a strictly subordinate position in the hierarchy. They became increasingly dedicated to their own field, ceasing to play any part in general medical care, but often actively proselytising wherever possible. Specialist societies formed sparingly in the nineteenth century but proliferated rapidly in the twentieth. At first, discussions were confined to clinical problems but as the fight for recognition went on, the organisation and expansion of the specialty became the major objective.

A striking feature of this history is that Britain lagged far behind Western Europe and North America in the development of clinical specialties. We are of course reluctant to take the view that this was simply a reflection of the backwardness of British medicine in general when some individual Britons have made important contributions to progress, but equally the claim that, by preserving the general approach, advances have been made more possible is unconvincing in view of the massive input from specialists elsewhere. It may be that the traditional British admiration for the gentleman amateur created as a corollary a disdain for the specialists, while the prestige of the two Royal Colleges dominated by the generalist and conservative establishments inhibited the development of newer disciplines. In other European countries, colleges had disappeared or lost influence by the eighteenth century, leaving the universities, with more diverse interests, as leaders in the medical field. Moreover the successful development of general practice and the referral system which was commonly adopted deprived the early specialists of the economic support inherent in the self referral practice common in Europe and North America. It is accepted wisdom that in Britain the special hospitals provided the springboard from which specialists achieved recognition and acceptability, but the course of events varied very remarkably between one specialty and another.

The specialist hospitals as we know them appeared first in the mid-eighteenth century and the earliest aimed to provide care for patients specifically excluded from the new general infirmaries. They were voluntary hospitals depending upon charitable support and were found therefore principally in prosperous centres where there was a long tradition of benevolence. London was in almost all cases the leader and in each specialty created a fashion which spread rapidly across the country. In the first phase were the lunatic hospitals, lying-in hospitals, houses of recovery for fevers and lock hospitals, obviously directed towards problems of wide public concern and later taken over by public provision. The second phase starting in the early nineteenth century produced a multitude of very small hospitals stimulated largely by professional interest, though again charitable support was always required and readily obtained. At the same time the crippled, the blind, the consumptives, and epileptics attracted considerable lay sympathy and benevolent institutions founded for their care and support were often later taken over by the doctors and converted into hospitals providing active treatment.

These small hospitals were very cheap to establish, though progressively more expensive to run. Many were started in private houses in areas of the city no longer fashionable. Some opened first as out-patient dispensaries, later acquiring a few beds and a resident matron. Except in the case of the lunatic hospitals the patients were all indigent refugees from appalling housing conditions and their hospital stay was prolonged. Almost all the hospitals had a chequered career. There were periods of financial crisis and defaulting hospital secretaries. The medical staff were often jealous, quarrelsome and at odds with the lay governors. Some closed with the death of their founder and others merged into larger institutions but many were saved from the brink of disaster by a new enthusiast amongst the doctors or the benefactors. Throughout this period intense hostility towards them was voiced in the professional journals but they were not deserted by the laity. The public always likes a specialist or even a quack. Those which prospered enlarged and took on assistant physicians and surgeons as well as resident medical staff, a most important step in ensuring a succession.

In time the hospital staff despite individual antipathies became a coherent group, a specialist association in embryo and a base from which the specialty expanded to invade the general hospitals. Postgraduate teaching was from a very early period advertised as a feature of all the larger institutions. British universities were always sparing in their creation of professorial chairs but, when the time came, the concentration of clinical material and expertise of the specialist hospitals made them the obvious situation for the development of specialist clinical academic departments. The practical value of gathering together the sufferers from particular problems was well recognised during both World Wars. Orthopaedics, plastic surgery and neurosurgery all obtained an enormous impetus from the war time development of special units.

Obstetrics and Gynaecology

Since the lying-in hospitals were among the first to appear we may look briefly at the development of these two related specialties. In the late seventeenth and early eighteenth century, the management of obstetrics previously left to the midwives was increasingly engaging the interest of surgeons and man-midwives. Germany and France were well ahead of England in this respect, though the Chamberlen family with their secret development of the obstetric forceps were pioneers. It may be disputed as to what extent the invention of the forceps stimulated the interest of the growing body of surgeon apothecaries, but it would be surprising if it was not a factor.

In England William Giffard was the first after the Chamberlens to use them successfully in 1726, and Edward Chapman the first to give a published description in 1733 when he set up a school of midwifery in Red Lion Square in London. William Smellie (1697-1763) has some claim to be called the father of British obstetrics. Originally practising as a GP in Lanark he read of the forceps and came to London and subsequently Paris but returned to London in 1739 to set up a school of midwifery for surgeons and for midwives, demonstrating at deliveries in the patients' own homes. His lectures were published in 1742, 1748 and 1753 together with a valuable treatise and anatomical tables. He devised his own short forceps made in wood but used them sparingly and his example led to the conservative approach of English midwifery. It was however, William Hunter, his pupil who introduced a more scientific approach and established the reputation of the specialty, though he was in violent dispute with the College of Physicians. His book on the anatomy of the gravid uterus in 1774 is one of the classics. He was followed by Denman who continued his school, and by Osborne, Burton and Pugh in a period when England led the field in this branch of medicine and when it could first be said that a specialty existed.

It was in this period that the lying-in hospitals first appeared. In Dublin in 1745 the hospital which was subsequently the Rotunda was established in Bartholomew Mosse and set the trend. The British Lying-in Hospital was founded in Brownlow Street in 1749, the City of London Lying-in for Married Women in 1750, the General Lying-in (subsequently Queen Charlotte's) in 1752, the Newcastle Lying-in (subsequently Princess Mary's) 1760, the General Lying-in Hospital (subsequently the New Westminster) 1765, the Manchester Lying-in (subsequently St Mary's) 1790, Edinburgh 1793, Belfast 1794.

Except for the last, which was the initiative of a clergyman, each of these special hospitals was set up by a medical man and each had as a primary object the training of midwives. They were also charitable institutions for the assistance of the poor and inadequately housed and for most the indications for admission were social rather than medical. The moral tone of charity also demanded that they were for married women, but some allowed the delivery of the first child of an unmarried mother much to the annoyance of the parochial authorities who had to shoulder the financial burden of bastards.

The turnover of patients was very slow. They might be in for two or three weeks before and again after delivery. There was no resident medical staff but usually a matron. The medical management varied considerably. At the Rotunda the Master appeared to have exercised a strong authority, and in the New Westminster Dr John Leake produced an important text book based on his experience but elsewhere there seems to have been less involvement. William Hunter and Sandys were both on the staff of the British Hospital, though the fearsome incidence of puerperal fever led them to distance themselves a little, while the General Lying-in, after a fine start under Sir Richard Manningham, ran down very seriously in a succession of moves until it was resuscitated in the nineteenth century under Queen Charlotte's patronage.

As so often with the special hospitals, in Manchester the establishment of the Lying-in Hospital resulted primarily from dissension amongst the staff of the Infirmary. Charles White, a surgeon and man-midwife who had been a pioneer in hygienic management and author of an influential *Treatise on the Management of Lying-in Women* had been one of the founders of the Infirmary from which pregnant women were excluded. The new hospital was intended for the training of midwives. It started with a few beds but was largely an outpatient and district service and for a time ran so short of funds that the beds closed altogether. Elsewhere lying-in charities rather than hospitals were founded in many towns and cities.

The establishment of these special hospitals in the eighteenth century was a manifestation of medical interest in midwifery but they did not immediately become the training ground for specialist obstetricians or the focal point for development of the discipline as did hospitals in other specialties. There were to begin with no medical residents to maintain the succession. Obstetrics was taught in private schools, or it was not taught at all. Edinburgh led the way by appointing a "City Professor" Joseph Gibson in 1726 for the proper education of midwives. The third holder of this office in 1756 obtained beds in the Royal Infirmary for the instruction of medical students but other city centres were far behind.

No doubt all provincial surgeons, who were for the substantial part of their time general practitioners, were involved in obstetrics to some extent but it seems likely that in large towns and cities some became recognised informally as specialists in the field. We have however little record of their activities. In Liverpool Henry Park is reported to have delivered 4,000 children between 1769 and 1830, John McCulloch, 4,832 between 1797 and 1820. More remarkable however was Edward Rigby (1747-1821) born in Manchester but apprenticed to Martineau, a surgeon in Norwich; before the age of thirty he had produced an *Essay on Uterine Haemorrhage* defining the distinction between accidental and inevitable which was a masterpiece of observation. He was appointed to the staff of the Norfolk and Norwich Hospital and practiced surgery as well as obstetrics. He did not take a medical degree until he was 67 years of age. A remarkable man in many ways, he introduced a programme of vaccination in 1805, became Mayor of Norwich and fathered quadruplets when he was 70. In the provinces the distinction between surgeon and physician was never so sharp as in London but physicians always had higher status. The MD degree could be obtained with little more than a payment of a fee to some Scottish Universities and the senior surgeons were apt therefore to be remustered as physicians later in their careers. John Burton was one of the founders of the York Hospital in 1740 and its first physician but was also a writer on obstetrics.

The struggle by obstetricians for professional recognition and for an adequate training for all doctors is a sorry tale of obstruction by the two English Colleges, which we need not detail here.

By the mid-nineteenth century a new factor was beginning to emerge, gynaecological surgery. Some of the lying-in hospitals also catered for diseases of women. The Manchester hospital was reopened in 1854 as the Hospital and Dispensary for Diseases Peculiar to Women and Diseases of Children Under the Age of Six Years. However this did not necessarily imply much in the way of operative surgery. Vaginal discharge and misplacement of the uterus treated by douches and pessaries must have accounted for most of the business, though carcinoma of the cervix was treated by various cauterizing agents and menorrhagia by injecting fused potash into the uterus. Such patients were numerous, little provision was made for them in general hospitals and at least in London the lying-in hospitals would not take them. In 1842 Dr Protheroe Smith, Assistant Lecturer at Barts, and a group of sympathizers started the Hospital for Diseases of Women in 1843, first in Red Lion Square and subsequently in Soho Square. He was appointed as its first surgeon but two years later took his MD and was promoted to physician leaving Sanderson as surgeon and over the ensuing years the business of the hospital became increasingly surgical.

The ovarian cyst was the commonest and most readily removable abdominal tumour and had tempted surgeons from a very early period. In the north, Charles Clay established abdominal operations as practicable even without anaesthesia. In Manchester he performed his first ovariotomy in 1842 and a hysterectomy in 1844. After the introduction of anaesthesia the number of operations went up dramatically. He is believed to have carried out 400 ovariotomies with an overall mortality of 25%. He demonstrated his method to Spencer Wells who made operative gynaecology the growing edge of the surgery. Clay was briefly attached to the St Mary's Hospital in Manchester but most of his work was carried out in private. He left however a tradition in the hospital taken up by Lloyd Roberts one of the most famous gynaecologists in the north who defined his speciality "as anything curable or lucrative".

In London the Samaritan Hospital was founded in 1847 but was not really active until Spencer Wells came back from the Crimean War and together with Baker Brown embarked on ovariotomy. He soon demonstrated that his technique and perhaps his attention to cleanliness could reduce mortality progressively. In 1877 he published results; Guy's Hospital mortality 52.43%, Hospital for Women Soho Square 38.16%, Samaritan 23.84%. These special hospitals achieved a place in the specialty which was never reached by the lying-in hospitals. Spencer Wells was never on the staff of any general hospital yet he was world famous with an enormous practice and became

President of the Royal College of Surgeons. The trend was not confined to London. Lawson Tait, a brilliant if aggressive young surgeon trained in Edinburgh, did his first ovariotomy when a house surgeon in Wakefield in 1868, and moved to Birmingham Hospital for Diseases of Women in 1871 of which he was first surgeon. He rivalled Spencer Wells' records and considerably enlarged the scope of operative abdominal gynaecology, going on later to undertake upper abdominal surgery pioneering cholecystectomy. Again he was on the staff of no other hospital though accorded the title of Professor of Gynaecology at Queen's College in 1887.

There could however be antagonism between the infirmary general surgeons and those in special hospitals. In Liverpool Francis Imlach trained as a surgeon in the lying-in hospital. He was appointed to the Women's Hospital in 1882 and embarked on operative treatment, particularly of the uterine appendages for which he was pilloried and ruined by his professional colleagues.

James Aveling is remarkable in having founded two special hospitals: the first in 1865, the Sheffield Hospital for Women, subsequently endowed by Thomas Jessop, the second in 1871, the Chelsea Hospital for Women. This hospital played and still plays an important part in the development of gynaecology. John Bland Sutton was appointed to the surgical staff of the Middlesex in 1886 but had no beds. He was largely concerned with pathology. In 1895 he was appointed to Chelsea and remained there until 1910 when he became PRCS. It was at Chelsea that he worked out the technique which made hysterectomy a safe operation and established his enormous practice. Victor Bonney, one of his successors at both hospitals had the experience of working out his advances at Chelsea before assuming senior status at the Middlesex Hospital at the age of 58.

Obstetrics and gynaecology are now grouped together as one specialty and practiced in every district hospital. Obstetrics for the younger, gynaecology for the older members, but as we have seen the origins were somewhat different. The lying-in hospitals were amongst the first specialist hospitals but were basically incidental to the development of the specialty which had a century in which to struggle to gain acceptability. Gynaecological surgery from its base in special hospitals was influential to surgery in general and became an indispensable part of every general hospital.

Psychiatry

Much has been written on the history of psychiatry, though little of it apart from the writings of Hunter and McAlpine on its development as a professional specialty in Britain. To those nourished on the cartoon character beside the analyst's couch it comes as a surprise to learn that in this country specialist psychiatry was in origin almost exclusively hospital based.

The lunatic hospitals and asylums were among the first special hospitals and became by far the largest and most numerous. In the early eighteenth century there was the endowed Bethlem Hospital in London and rather remarkably the Bethel Hospital in Norwich founded by charity in 1713. The new phase opened with the establishment of St Luke's Hospital in London in 1751, an independent voluntary hospital, and the lunatic hospitals in Manchester, Liverpool, York, Newcastle and Exeter, which were all attached to or at least under the control of the general infirmary of those cities. They were of course places of confinement for psychotics, particularly the violent, and such medical treatment as was administered was simply "lowering" by purges and emetics. The general physicians with oversight of these hospitals, such as Dr Arnold of Leicester and Dr Haslam of the Bethlem, wrote treatises upon the nature of lunacy and the treatment of lunatics but would scarcely be considered psychiatrists in the modern sense. Often the medical men with charge of the numerous private mad houses had more intimate knowledge of the management, as for instance Dr Willis who was called in to help with George III's problem. But conditions in many of these places were outrageous and the Visitation by the Royal College of Physicians never more than perfunctory. Exposure of the scandalous cruelty and neglect in many of the lunatic hospitals called out for reform. Slowly after the Act of 1808 and rapidly after the Act of 1845, the county asylums were established, away from the city

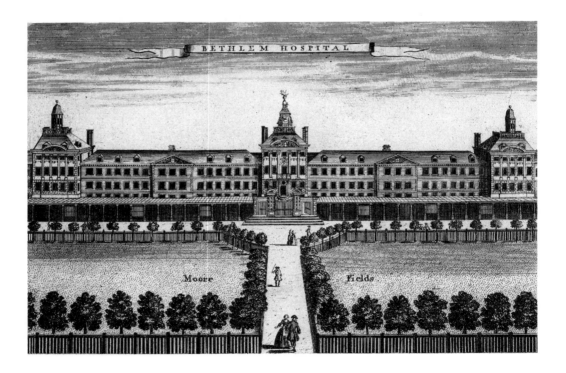

4 . Bethlem Hospital in the 18th century. The hospital later moved to a new building in Lambeth, now used as the Imperial War Museum.

centre and away from the control of the infirmary physicians. Increasingly they were staffed by medical men, usually with the minimum qualifications, who were resident, poorly paid, forbidden private practice or out-patient consultation and (in spite of the respect accorded to some such as John Connolly) of low status.

The first professional association was formed in 1841 - the Association of Medical Officers of Asylums and Hospitals for the Insane. This organisation became in 1865 the Medico Psychological Association and ultimately the Royal College of Psychiatrists. It was the body officially consulted by the Profession and ran a Postgraduate Diploma in psychological medicine between 1886 and 1911, when some universities were induced to set up their own diploma. The first Journal, started by the Medical Superintendent of the Devon County Asylum in 1854, was the *Asylum Journal of Mental Science* although later the word asylum was dropped from the title.

By 1900 there were some fifteen large asylums in the London area and 89 in the rest of England, employing a very large number of doctors, who were however confined in their work to the psychotics and to hospitals increasingly over-crowded by chronic cases. The neuroses received little attention from the medical profession. There was never in England any development of neuro-psychiatry as there was under Charcot in Paris and when Elliotson as Professor of Medicine at UCH toyed with hypnotism he was quickly evicted from his post. The fervour and excitement created by Freud and his contemporaries in Vienna left England largely untouched and although the message was brought here by Ernest Jones it had little impact on the professional body. Although there was some useful neuro-pathology undertaken in some asylums, the Royal in Edinburgh, the West Riding and at Claybury by Frederick Mott, the second half of the nineteenth century saw British psychiatry stultified by its confinement to the asylums. The revival after the First World War started with the opening of the Maudsley Hospital specifically reserved for acute cases and by the leadership of Aubrey Lewis, Dean of the Institute of Psychiatry, who subsequently inspired the medical schools to take up the academic study of the problem but it was only after the Second World War that British psychiatry achieved the status and vigour which it now enjoys.

Ophthalmology

Ophthalmology was the first branch of surgery to obtain recognition as a specialty, to establish its own professional institutions, and to achieve exclusive control of its field. It was heavily dependent in its early stages upon the special hospitals. 1805, when Saunders founded the hospital which later became known as Moorfields, is generally regarded as the starting point. There is justification for this view in respect of the qualified medical profession but it is important to set this development in a broader context. Itinerant oculists were practising in England from at least the early sixteenth century. They had a capacity for salesmanship, a certain dexterity but very little or no theoretical training. Most of their treatment consisted in the application of drops and of ointment, but cataract was a common affliction in all parts of the known world and couching, displacing the opaque lens out of the axis of vision, was a surgical technique widely practised in Europe and the East from a very early period and was part of the stock in trade of the oculists.

The conventional medical profession was inclined to leave the eye problems to these oculists, some of whom attained positions of prominence. Samuel Pepys had cause to attend one but was later perturbed to discover his ignorance. "Strange he said that this Turberville should be so great a man yet to this day had seen no eye dissected". Although some surgeons throughout the eighteenth century would undertake cataract operations they devoted little study to the problems of the eye and a remarkable succession of oculists obtained Court Appointments. William Read who attended Queen Anne was knighted: he was succeeded by Grant, a one-eyed former cobbler. The Chevalier Taylor, who travelled Europe claiming to be Ophthalmiator Pontifical and Imperial, was oculist to George I and obtained Royal Appointments for his son and grandson. In spite of his razzmatazz, Taylor made a significant contribution to the surgery of squint.

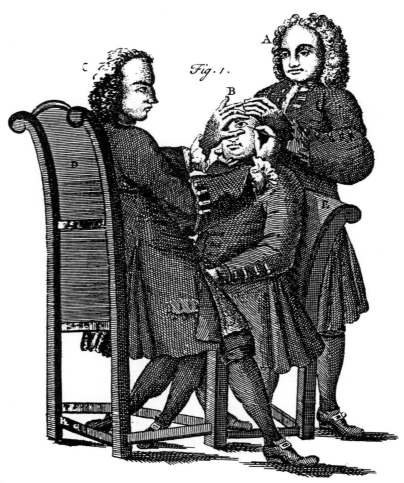

5. Couching a cataract.

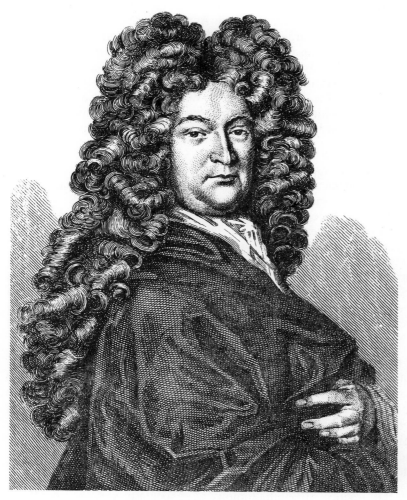

6.
Sir William Read,
oculist to Queen
Anne.

Meanwhile on the Continent, particularly in Germany, there was more scientific study. Boerhaave of Leyden wrote a treatise on the pathology of the eye. In France, Daviel devised the operation for extraction of cataract in 1745 and in Vienna a school of ophthalmology was established in 1773 by Joseph Bath, whose successors as professors of ophthalmic medicine in the university attracted students from all over Europe. In England Dr Wathen, oculist to George III, revived some interest by his book on theory of cataract in 1785 but tradition has it that the return of British troops from Egypt in 1803 brought to England very many sufferers from purulent ophthalmia and trachoma which then spread to the local population and this epidemic alerted the English medical profession to the problems of eye disease.

This no doubt set the scene but it was not the whole story. Saunders, a protégé of Astley Cooper, was deemed ineligible for a surgical appointment at Guy's, and determined therefore to make his own way by a new venture, the Dispensary for the Poor Afflicted with Diseases of the Eye and the Ear founded in 1805. As a first step he secured the written approval of all the physicians and surgeons of both Guys and St Thomas's - he had to demonstrate that ophthalmology was a proper subject for the fully trained and qualified surgeon; that was perhaps his most important step. The Dispensary soon became a hospital and the patients flocked in although there was an almost simultaneous foundation of the Royal Infirmary for the Diseases of the Eye by Wathen in Cork Street. Saunders had soon to abandon the ear which "was laborious but led neither to distinction nor obtained even the common reward of benevolent institutions". It was an experience to be repeated elsewhere.

Saunders' Foundation was very rapidly followed by the establishment of Eye Hospitals all over the country - eighteen outside and four more inside London in thirty years. Some were founded by his own pupils, the first by William Adams in Exeter in 1808. Saunders himself died young but his successors Travers and Lawrence, having both made contributions to ophthalmology, returned in their later years to the practice of general surgery at Guy's and at Bart's. William Goldwyer who founded the Bristol Eye Hospital in 1810 called himself at first surgeon and oculist but later dropped the term oculist in case it was thought that he was exclusively concerned with eye disease. William James Wilson, a pupil of Saunders, founded the Manchester Institution for Curing Diseases of the Eye in 1813 when he found there was no way of getting on the staff of the Infirmary in that city, but when such an opportunity did appear in 1827 he resigned from the Eye Hospital.

For the first half of the nineteenth century ophthalmology was recognised as a specialty but only as a part time interest and not one from which to reach the pinnacle of the profession. The hospitals were easy to establish and cheap, most of the patients were ambulant, few were mortally ill. They had shown that ophthalmology was properly a part of conventional medicine and that there was an enormous reservoir of patients formerly left to the unqualified. Curiously neither the ophthalmologists at this stage nor their predecessors, the oculists, were seriously concerned with spectacles, the haphazard sale of which they left to shopkeepers and itinerants.

By the mid-century the practice of ophthalmology as a specialty was secure. Some surgeons continued to practice general surgery as well but no longer so readily abandoned their Eye Hospital appointment. The decade 1850-60 was remarkable in that ophthalmology then first achieved its international reputation. William Bowman at Moorfields undertook fundamental physiological studies which gave surgical practice a scientific basis; Von Helmholz discovered the ophthalmoscope in 1851, although his work had been foreshadowed in London by William Cumming; Franz Donders in Holland brought in the practice of refraction; Von Graefe from Germany published his work on glaucoma, and all this group came together at an Ophthalmological Congress in 1857. By this time Guy's, UCH and St Mary's had all appointed ophthalmic surgeons to their own specialist departments but in London, Moorfields Hospital which had grown steadily after a series of moves held pride of place and the first English journal to be published was *The Ophthalmic Hospital Reports* from 1857. The Ophthalmic Society of the United Kingdom was founded in 1880 and in the same year there was an Ophthalmic Section at the BMA Annual Meeting with requests to the GMC to require undergraduate instruction and appropriate examination questions as part of the qualifying examination.

In spite of the acceptance by General Hospitals of ophthalmic departments, existing Eye Hospitals thrived and new ones were founded, though now of course by eye surgeons already trained in that discipline. Thus in 1889 Mr John Bullar having been Ophthalmic House Surgeon at Barts and obtained his FRCS moved to Southampton and set up the Free Eye Hospital there, initially at his own expense. By the turn of the century, recognised ophthalmologists monopolised the consulting practice in eye disorders and have since achieved a very considerable material prosperity.

Orthopaedics

Orthopaedics as a surgical specialty in Britain evolved from two schools in London and Liverpool, each with a strong special hospital focus which were brought together by the genius, and geniality of one man, Robert Jones, in the specialist military hospital set up during the First World War. There was of course a long non-surgical background, concerned on the one hand with charitable care of the crippled child and on the other with the tradition of manipulation derived from the bone setters, while there was a major input into relevant surgical technique by the master general surgeons of the late nineteenth century.

The London story starts with W.J. Little, who suffered himself from clubbing of the foot and although anxious to pursue a career as a physician was determined to explore the surgical possibility of the cure of his own deformity. He visited Louis Stromeyer in Hanover, who successfully performed a subcutaneous tenotomy of his *tendo achilles* to very good effect; the system was extensively taken up in Germany and France and Little returned to England, brought together his friends and patrons to found in 1840 the Orthopaedic Institution in Bloomsbury Square, subsequently the Royal Orthopaedic Hospital. Little himself having acquired an MRCP was physician, his brother-in-law Tamplin the surgeon. The latter was unfortunately a jealous and quarrelsome man, determined to monopolise the treatment and Little subsequently withdrew. Tamplin also quarrelled with an assistant surgeon, Chance, and as a result another orthopaedic hospital, The City of London was founded in 1851, at which Chance remained sole surgeon until he was 86 years of age. Happily the treatment seems to have been predominantely non-surgical. Then in 1864 the Society for Diseases of the Spine and Hips was transmogrified into the National Orthopaedic Hospital, Bolsover Street. The three hospitals all teetered on the brink of bankruptcy and the surgeons quarrelled with administrators and with one another, but the orthopaedic tradition of long term treatment of deformities by splints, braces and supports together with occasional tenotomy was established and some of the surgeons also obtained appointments at the more progressive teaching hospitals.

Then with the new era in surgery started by Lister there was an immediate widening of scope. William McEwen the Glasgow general surgeon, established from 1880 onwards the value of osteotomy for deformities and Arbuthnot Lane at Guy's and Great Ormond Street brought in the no touch technique and the plating of fractures.   These new initiatives, together with the amalgamation (engineered by the King's Fund) of the three small orthopaedic hospitals finalised in 1907, gave a new impetus to the London School. The succession of resident house surgeons in the new hospital, Royal National Orthopaedic, established the pattern of specialist training. Harry Platt of Manchester was one of the first to serve.

Meanwhile in Liverpool, Hugh Owen Thomas from the fourth generation of a line of Welsh bone-setters but himself trained in traditional medicine had established in the 1860's a personal reputation for orthopaedic treatment largely by splinting and manipulation. Clearly he was a remarkable character, self reliant and anti-establishment but with real mechanical talent and clinical skill. He was the founder of the Liverpool school. In 1873 his nephew by marriage, Robert Jones, came to work with him and absorbing Thomas's teaching was able to fuse it with the surgical tradition of the conventional schools. He rapidly established his own reputation and in 1888 was appointed consulting surgeon to the Manchester Ship Canal. Shortly afterwards he was appointed to the Royal Southern Hospital and, in 1898, he was drawing up schemes for special hospitals for children with crippling diseases, many of whom suffered from tuberculosis and therefore required long term care, with rest, good food and country air. In 1900 the Royal Liverpool Country Hospital for Children, Hesswall, was opened with this remit, among the first of many country hospitals for orthopaedic cases which became a focus for development of the speciality.

About this time Jones also met, and treated, Agnes Hunt, a spirited girl of good family who herself suffered a crippling septic arthritis of the hip in childhood, running a small home and hospital at Baschurch in Shropshire for cripples. From 1903 Robert Jones attended there and shuttled cases back and forth from Liverpool. The hospital subsequently moved to Oswestry and achieved world fame as the Robert Jones and Agnes Hunt Orthopaedic Hospital. The need for country hospitals for children with bone and joint tuberculosis, osteomyelitis and polio as well as congenital deformities was becoming widely appreciated. The Heritage Craft School and subsequently hospital was set up at Chailey in 1903, the Lord Mayor Treloar Cripples Hospital and College was founded at Alton in 1908, St Gerrard's Hospital, Birmingham in 1912 and the Queen Mary's, Carshalton shortly afterwards.

Then came the War. Robert Jones, although not perhaps set in the accepted military mould, was the obvious person to organise the longer-term care of the injured and did so with great effect at the Shepherds Bush Military Hospital London and the Alder Hey Hospital, Liverpool. He gathered around him the younger elements from both the London and Liverpool schools and from this amalgamation the specifically British specialty of orthopaedics was born. His team included all the great names of post-war orthopaedics and since a number of American surgeons were also posted to Shepherds Bush he established a lasting trans-Atlantic liaison.

After the War the country hospitals multiplied. No less than 26 were started during the 20's and 30's: the Wingfield Hospital, Oxford; St Nicholas, Pyrford; The Royal

Orthopaedic, Birmingham (union of two earlier institutions); Wrightington in Lancashire; Black Knotley in Essex; Princess Margaret Rose in Edinburgh, to name but a few. The importance of the country branch was recognised by the teaching hospitals and the Stanmore Branch of the Royal National Orthopaedic Hospital was opened in 1922. The tempo of these places was leisurely, the children would be in for years so that they were schools as well as hospitals but they could draw their consultants from a wide area and it was possible for a London surgeon to be on the staff of Oswestry attending once a month for a concentrated weekend of consultation and operation. However at Stanmore the idea of having a senior surgeon permanently and exclusively on site gave an opportunity for detailed and prolonged observation. Fortunately they appointed Herbert Seddon to that post, who built up such a reputation for himself that shortly before the War he took the first Professorial Chair in orthopaedics, the Nuffield Chair in Oxford.

Meanwhile outside London orthopaedic surgeons were taking on the treatment of fractures - not without stubborn resistance from the general surgeons. Harry Platt in fact started a fracture clinic at Ancoats, Manchester before the First War, but it was many years before injuries were regarded as part of the orthopaedic surgeon's remit and Watson-Jones in Liverpool was probably the most influential in achieving this end. In the Second War Rowley Bristow from Pyrford and St Thomas's took over to good effect the role of his teacher Robert Jones, further emphasizing the vital role of orthopaedics in the treatment of injuries.

Nowadays orthopaedics is a part of every district service. Orthopaedic surgeons are almost as numerous as general surgeons and demarcation disputes are largely settled. Bone and joint tuberculosis, osteomyelitis and polio are almost things of the past and the country hospitals are now closing or being converted into other use or providing accommodation for hip replacement in the elderly. The Royal National Orthopaedic Hospital has closed its London Branch and been absorbed in the Middlesex. Looking back however it is clear that the special hospitals by building up their expertise in isolation were central to the development of the specialty in Britain.

Paediatrics

Children's hospitals are amongst the most widespread and most readily accepted of all the specialist hospitals. They proliferated rapidly in the 1850's and 60's yet paradoxically paediatrics scarcely existed as a specialty in Britain until after the First World War and did not thrive until after the Second.

Children under the age of six were from the start excluded from most general infirmaries. It was believed that they could not properly be separated from their mothers and a very high infant mortality was accepted as seemingly inevitable. It is extraordinary how slowly the profession acquired a concern for childhood disease and initially hospitalisation was scarcely even considered as a possibility. Armstrong's dispensary for children in Red Lion Square lasted no more than ten years in the 1760's. Rather more effectively John Bunnell Davis, part of whose medical education was in France, set up in 1816 a dispensary, which also flagged after his death in 1824 although it was ultimately reborn as the Royal Waterloo Hospital for Women and Children. In Manchester, the General Dispensary for Children operated from 1829 onwards but made little inroad into the formidable problem of infectious disease in childhood.

However from 1850 onwards the scene changed dramatically and almost simultaneously in a number of major cities, usually under the stimulus of the incidence of epidemic disease and its appalling mortality in children. In 1852 the Hospital for Sick Children, Great Ormond Street first opened its doors under the inspiration of Dr Charles West who had visited Paris and Berlin where there were already children's hospitals. In Manchester, Dr Louis Borchardt, an immigrant physician from Prussia joined the Dispensary there which by 1856 had changed its name and ultimately developed into the Pendlebury "Manchester Children's Hospital". Concurrently Dr August Merei, a Hungarian immigrant joined with James Whitehead, a surgeon to the Lying-in Hospital, to found the "Clinical Hospital for Diseases of Children". Incidentally, another Prussian, Abraham Jacobi, emigrated to the USA at the same time and rather rapidly stimulated the growth of American paediatrics.

Meanwhile Liverpool, where epidemic fevers were most prevalent, was the first city to appoint in 1848 a Medical Officer of Health, Dr W.H. Duncan, and in 1851 the Liverpool Institution for Diseases of Children was opened by Alfred Stevens, a surgeon, as a dispensary. It was converted into an infirmary with in-patients in 1856 ultimately to become the Royal Liverpool Children's Hospital. In Norwich the impetus came from the charitable laity and from J.G. Johnson, a surgeon at the Norfolk and Norwich, the money being raised by concerts given by Jenny Lind, and a converted house in Pottergate was opened as an infirmary in 1853. Leeds and Bristol both had children's hospitals in 1857, Edinburgh 1860, Birmingham and Newcastle 1862.

By 1900 no less than ten of the children's hospitals in London were largely staffed by physicians attached to the teaching hospitals. Elsewhere the usual pattern of staffing consisted of one or two general physicians and a rather large number of general practitioners enrolled as Medical Officers, "Surgeons" or Assistant Physicians. Yet the British contribution to the knowledge of childhood disease before the First War was miniscule.

Frederick Still in the first years of the twentieth century was the first physician to confine his practice to children but outside London there was no recognition of paediatrics until after the First World War. The British Paediatric Association was founded with six members in 1928 and did not achieve a membership of 500 until 1969. By contrast Bellevue Hospital in New York already had a Clinical Professor for the diseases of children in 1861. *The American Journal of Obstetrics and Diseases of Women and Children* was founded in 1869 and devoted most of its articles to the young. *The Archives of Paediatrics* was founded in 1884, the Journal *Paediatrics* in 1896, the *American Journal of Diseases of Childhood* 1911. In Germany the *Zeitung fur Kinderkrankheiten* commenced publication in 1843 and there were certainly professors in the 1880's.

Why it may then be asked did Britain lag behind? There was of course the general reluctance in this country to allow specialisation and the physicians were even more

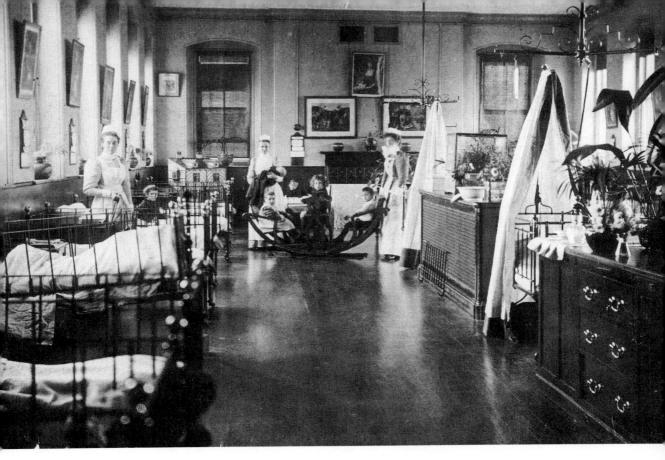

7. Childrens' ward in the Royal United Hospital, Bath. c1905.

resistant than the surgeons. In the early years scarlet fever, diphtheria and other epidemic infections made up the bulk of admissions presenting perhaps the general problems of fevers rather than the specific problems of childhood. Children under the age of two years were only admitted in the most exceptional circumstances so that the problems of infant feeding did not immediately impinge upon the physicians. In the larger hospitals the supervision was provided by younger physicians and surgeons whose chief objective was to get a place on the staff of the infirmary or teaching hospital and who would resign from "the kids" as soon as they achieved it. It seems there was insufficient private practice in paediatrics to support them. This applied even to some of the great names, like Thomas Barlow who did such important work at Great Ormond Street on scurvy, Garrod who worked on congenital metabolic disorders and many others. In the smaller hospitals care was largely in the hands of local GP's who saw it as but a small part of their practice, although interestingly enough in the USA almost all the pioneers of paediatrics started from the base of general practice.

When paediatrics did at last emerge it was very often based on the children's hospitals, although by the 20's and 30's most large hospitals had children's wards. Paediatricians now make a very large contribution to overall medical care (BPA now has 2,000 members) but it must remain something of an indictment of British medicine that the huge opportunities provided by the numerous children's hospitals were not exploited very much earlier.

Paediatric surgery was an even later development. The technical possibilities of the particular contribution of this group, the major surgery of the neonate, were not available until after the Second World War, while for older children the surgical field was already divided between system specialists. When it came, paediatric surgery was almost exclusively the business of larger children's hospitals; the teaching and larger general hospitals still fight a rear-guard action to resist it.

SUMMARY

The special hospitals were founded with varying motivation, professional or charitable, scientific or selfish: once in existence they provided remarkable opportunities for the study of disease and the applications of advances, and thus for the development of clinical specialty. Different groups made different uses, good and bad, of these opportunities. Many of the hospitals have now disappeared but the larger ones which remain have made outstanding contribution to practice, to teaching and to research and they are now demonstrating not simply the merits of specialisation but the potentiality of sub-specialisation in their discipline.

A select bibliography will be provided by the author on request.

ON THE TRACK OF WOOZLES: Where was the first Cottage Hospital?

R Meyrick Emrys-Roberts

"The tracks!" said Pooh. *"A third animal has joined the other two!"* [1]

John R Guy recently wrote an essay-review of nine hospital histories. He chose for his title: "Of the writing of hospital histories there is no end" [2]

One reason for this glut is the number of centenary celebrations amongst cottage hospitals, two of which were covered by John Guy's review, one at Halstead in Essex, the other at Butleigh, a village near Glastonbury in Somerset. Note that I class these two with confidence as Cottage hospitals; both were started in 1880. I have less confidence about another village hospital in John Guy's list. In this case the foundation was very much earlier, at Wiveliscombe, a few miles west of Taunton. Here, in 1804, the energetic and reputedly eccentric village surgeon, Dr Henry Sully, converted a small house into a dispensary, mainly for out-patients but with a bed or two for the more seriously sick. His financial backer and encourager was a local brewer, William Hancock. For about eight years Wiveliscombe Dispensary and Infirmary was the only voluntary hospital between Exeter and Bath. Dr Sully's enthusiasm attracted notice elsewhere and by 1825 there were medical students in attendance, and the little hospital counted among its consultants the famous and ubiquitous Sir Astley Cooper, doyen of London surgeons. But the scale of work remained modest, and eventually the building was used as surgery accommodation for local GP's, who were seeing patients there as recently as 1985.

Was Wiveliscombe Dispensary and Infirmary the first Cottage Hospital? As far as I know it has never staked such a claim, unlike at least three other buildings in England. One of these is part of a row of cottages on the outskirts of Hemel Hempstead in Hertfordshire. Above the door is a handsome plaque carrying the words:

IN THIS ROW OF COTTAGES
SIR ASTLEY COOPER BART SURGEON
TO KING GEORGE IV, SENIOR SURGEON
AT GUY's HOSPITAL 1800 TO 1825
OPENED THE FIRST COTTAGE HOSPITAL
JANUARY 1827

This cottage at Piccott's End is well worth a visit, if only to see some very remarkable mediaeval wall-paintings, which were revealed by chance a few years ago. I would hesitate, however, to commend a special visit for pilgrims worshipping the site of the first cottage hospital. Agreed - it was a hospital in a cottage, but was it ever a cottage hospital? In view of the problems of definition this decision has to be a matter of interpretation or semantics. It was created more for the personal advantage of Sir Astley Cooper than for the local residents, - initially, anyway. Sir Astley, trying to escape from the exigencies of popularity in London had retreated to Gadebridge, an estate on the borders of Hemel

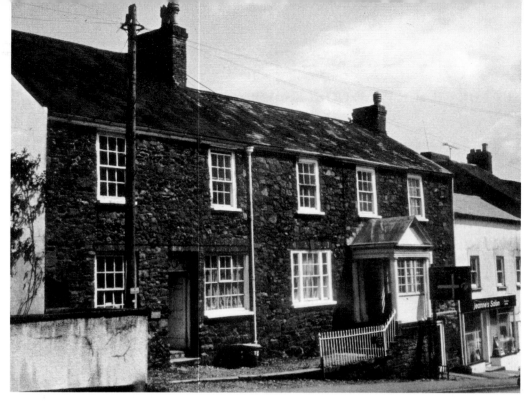

8. The Wiveliscombe Dispensary and Infirmary, founded 1804.

9. (below). The first Wincanton Cottage Hospital, opened in 1900. It had two wards, each with three beds. The hospital moved to larger premises in 1920.

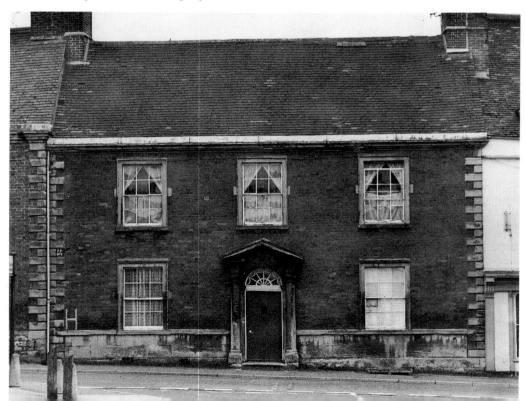

Hempstead where he had ambitions to become a gentleman-farmer in semi-retirement.[3] But persistent patients followed him there, and the hospital was opened as a means of meeting their demands. To obtain help he enlisted two local practitioners as honorary surgeons, but the little hospital was inadequate and within four years a new and sizeable hospital had been built by a benefactor on another site. This subsequently developed into today's West Herts Hospital.

If Sir Astley Cooper's foundation at Hemel Hempstead *was* a cottage hospital how should we classify the earliest phase of Salisbury Infirmary? In 1766 a row of houses in Fisherton Street was taken over "for the Relief of the Sick and Lame Poor". Simple furniture was installed and a Matron appointed and, with the aid of two nurses, the first patients were treated in April 1767. Meanwhile work had begun to prepare the new Infirmary which was to open in August 1771. Variations on this pattern can be found in the history of many voluntary hospitals, as for instance, the London Hospital. I doubt very much if any of these make-shift conversions would have been at any time called cottage hospitals although they were undoubtedly hospitals in cottages.

Another factor is the definition of a cottage. Could a small but tall town house qualify? Such a one, in Fenkel Street, Alnwick (in Northumberland) opened its doors to patients in 1819. In this house a room was supplied for the surgeon, another for the physician, one for the apothecary and another for the nurse - what a splendid example of early professional integration! Alnwick remained a fairly small market town and therefore the infirmary has never developed into a full-scale district hospital. Instead it has gradually grown to become one of the large cottage hospitals (or community hospitals to use the term of today) with a wide range of services supplied by local GPs and a number of visiting consultants.

In very much the same way the county hospital at Denbigh which started life in a rather grand building in 1807 has remained a microcosm of hospital care, being eventually refurbished as a community hospital in 1985 with fifty beds. For many years this much-loved hospital had been known affectionately by the local people as "the Cottage".

Any one of these early foundations could if they wished claim the credit of being the first cottage hospital; there are more to come. I am reminded of the chapter in Winnie-the-Pooh where Pooh-bear and Piglet go hunting. Walking round in circles in the snow they track their own foot-steps, deciding, as the tracks increase in number that they are on the path of Woozles. Meanwhile Christopher Robin, sitting on the branch of a tree above them can see the whole exercise in perspective.

Pooh and Piglet stopped anxiously when the number of tracks had grown to four. In the tracing of cottage hospitals we can find very many more. For instance, in 1818, in the village of Southam in Warwickshire the parish surgeon, Henry Lilley Smith,[4] opened a dispensary for the families of manual labourers. It was in an eight-roomed cottage and had four beds. No less than 305 patients are reported to have been admitted in the first fourteen months of its history. From the start the patients were expected to contribute towards their care, a novel system at a time when voluntary hospitals were expected to provide their services free. Adjoined to the hospital was an eye and ear dispensary and for many years sufferers from these types of condition received priority, until May 1860 when the premises were bought from Henry Smith's widow and beds were once again made available to all the local population. The matter of payment by patients was to become a salient issue in the cottage hospital movement, so Henry Smith's initiative is of special interest. The twentieth annual report of Southam Hospital states that for the first nineteen years the board was at the rate of 6s for men and 5s for women per week, with slightly lower rates for children. The impact of these charges on the labouring man can be appreciated when we consider that agricultural wages were in the neighbourhood of 10s per week. But at least the hospital soon became solvent, and remained so.

Details of Southam Hospital and about seventy others are contained in Chapter VII of a remarkable book published in 1870, entitled *Handybook of Cottage Hospitals*. The author, Dr Horace Swete, himself had established a hospital in the village of Wrington, (which lies in the Mendip Hills about twenty miles from Bath), in the year 1864. His interest in the subject of cottage hospitals was boundless, his style fluent and simple, and his range of aspect infinite, ranging from details of equipment and the correct attitude of the nursing staff to what he felt were the ideal flowers for the garden, "bright and sweet-scented and old-fashioned such as sweet briar, marjoram, boy's love, roses and bright scarlet geraniums". There should, he felt, be a settle by the fire for convalescing patients; the best colour for the walls should be warm buff; the best type of bed was Allen's patent, as shown at the Great Exhibition of 1851; children's cots should be as used in Great Ormond Street, fitted with a hinged side. He illustrates an ambulance which he designed himself and offers ideal plans for future cottage hospitals.

Horace Swete's *Handybook*, in my opinion, is more comprehensive than Florence Nightingale's *Notes on Hospitals* and *Notes on Nursing* put together. He collected details of every known foundation up to 1870, and was himself keen to establish the whereabouts of the first cottage hospital. Here he confused the issue by referring to two types hospital - village hospitals, and cottage hospitals which, he felt, were somewhat larger, with twelve to twenty beds. He gives as examples of the latter those at Middlesborough, North Ormesby, Marske, Stockton, Darlington, Hartlepool and Weston-super-Mare, nearly all of which, as you will have noticed, are in the neighbourhood of factories and iron-works. Yet all the hospitals he lists and describes come under his general title of *Cottage Hospitals*.

It is at Middlesborough that we can find another strong contender for the honour of being the first cottage hospital; rather surprisingly, perhaps, when cottage hospitals are generally thought of as being deep in the countryside. The main factor, however leading to their establishment is not rurality but isolation - distance from the nearest county or other voluntary hospital. In many areas such as Middlesborough, the Industrial Revolution had nurtured new towns in what were previously areas with scanty population.

The nearest hospital to Middlesborough in 1858 was at Newcastle some forty miles away. In that year a violent boiler explosion was to occur at the works of Messrs Snowdon and Hopkins which suddenly lit up the gross inadequacies of the medical services.[5]

To rectify the situation a local printer named John Jordison set off for the neighbouring town of Coatham and sought out a Miss Frances Mary Rachel Jacques, who was of the

Christ Church Sisterhood, and known to have received training as a nurse under Pastor Fliedner at the Deaconess Institute at Kaiserswerth near Düsseldorf. She responded promptly by renting with her own money two workmen's cottages, Nos 46 and 48 Dundas Mews, Middlesborough, and converting them to provide hospital accommodation at a cost of £181: too late, unfortunately, for the victims of the boiler explosion. The first patient, a Mr John McNally, severely injured in a drunken brawl, was admitted on March 7th 1859, just seven months ahead of Albert Napper's first patients in Cranleigh. The term cottage hospital seems to have been used from the start by those responsible for Middlesborough's first hospital.

The value of Sister Mary's creation was self-evident, but the cottages too small and uncomfortably hot, so plans were soon a foot for a purpose-built replacement, this time at the nearby town of North Ormesby because of the prohibitive cost of building-land in Middlesborough itself. The foundation stone was laid as early as July 9th 1860, and the new hospital opened on May 23rd 1861, a substantial building with, according to Horace Swete, no less than 28 beds, staffed by members of the Sisterhood and partly supported by a 1d per week scheme from the workers. One of the cottages in Dundas Mews was retained as a centre for out-patient work.

The people of Middlesborough claim 46 and 48 Dundas Mews as the site of England's first cottage hospital, but the people of Hemel Hempstead are equally convinced that Piccotts End should hold the title. So what are we to make of the plaque which can be found at the entrance to today's hospital at Cranleigh in Surrey? The wording used is:

CRANLEIGH VILLAGE HOSPITAL

THIS PART OF THE BUILDING WAS THE FIRST
VILLAGE HOSPITAL IN ENGLAND
FOUNDED IN THE YEAR 1859 BY
MR ALBERT NAPPER, SURGEON OF CRANLEIGH

The actual building stands alone, little changed since Albert Napper's day, a small cottage half-timbered and tile-hung in the style so common in Surrey, and thought to be some 500 years old. The moment that precipitated its conversion into a hospital is described by Swete in his *Handybook*. The rector of Cranleigh the Revd J.H. Sapte had been extremely concerned about the plight of the sick poor for some time and one day in the autumn of 1859 was riding across the common to discuss his ideas with some of his parishioners, "when he happened to hear that a severe accident had occurred and that the poor sufferer had been carried into the nearest cottage. Hastening thither he found Mr Napper (sic) with the assistance of his dispenser, the policeman, and an old woman (the druggist had offered his help, but had fainted and was useless) engaged in amputating the poor man's thigh". Mr Sapte at once placed at Mr Napper's disposal a small cottage rent-free which, after being white-washed and simply furnished was in a few weeks opened (and here I am using Swete's actual words) "as the first *Cottage Hospital*".

The total cost of conversion was less than £70. The brick-paved ground floor provided a kitchen, store-room and sitting-room. Upstairs were two wards of two beds, a nurse's room and an operating-room which could house two extra beds when necessary. The hospital was opened in October 1859 and by the end of 1863 had received 100 in-patients, approximately half of which could be classified as surgical. Amongst those seriously injured were four navvies, a bargeman, and a railway labourer. It was not only agricultural labourers that were the main accident victims in isolated parts of rural Britain. The countryside was being invaded by the work-gangs and machinery needed first to dig the canals and then to lay the railways. And there were, of course numerous coal-mines, copper and tin mines, slate quarries and china-clay workings in rural areas. So the prime essential for the country doctor was to be a skilled surgeon.

Albert Napper of Cranleigh was just such a man. His primary training at St Thomas' Hospital had been augmented by studying at Edinburgh and Bonn, and before moving to Cranleigh he had gained sixteen valuable years of experience in Guildford. Not only was his reputation as a practical surgeon excellent, but he was a thinking and methodical man, and kept careful records of his patients. Above all he was deeply interested in every aspect of their welfare. The founding of his hospital soon became known about elsewhere and just five months after its opening, on March 3rd 1860, the *British Medical Journal* devoted a leader to his work. "We commend the scheme to the notice of our associates in rural districts. The principle is excellent ... It brings the blessings of hospital accommodation home to the door of the villager ... and gives the provincial surgeon the means of making himself equal to all the emergencies which may occur in his profession."

Such publicity brought enquiries and visitors from all parts of Britain and a band of enthusiastic followers began to set up similar hospitals in their own villages. Early among these was Dr John Moore of Bourton-on-the-Water who opened a 6-bedded hospital on the Cranleigh model on March 11th 1861, and Dr John Henry Rogers who started a hospital in East Grinstead on October 14th 1863 in a tile-hung cottage, to which two more rooms had been added, mostly at his own expense. By curious coincidence East Grinstead was the home town of a Revd C W Payne-Crawfurd who had been the Rector of Bourton-on-the-Water and a close collaborator with Dr Moore in the preparations for opening his hospital.[6]

The conjunction of priest and doctor as prime movers in the establishment of cottage hospitals was to become a regular feature of earlier foundations. Very few hospitals of this sort were set up by religious orders such as the Sisters of Mercy, and, to the best of my belief, there was no movement in the Church to found hospitals on a par with that of Church of England schools.

To meet the demand for information (and inspiration) on the subject Albert Napper wrote a paper which was first published in a new monthly serial *The Medical Mirror* and subsequently in a pamphlet published by H.K. Lewis in 1864. I will give its title in full because of its implications:

ON
THE ADVANTAGES DERIVABLE
TO THE
MEDICAL PROFESSION AND THE PUBLIC
FROM
THE ESTABLISHMENT
OF
VILLAGE HOSPITALS
WITH
GENERAL INSTRUCTIONS CONCERNING COSTS, PLANS, RULES,
AND AN APPROPRIATE DIETARY
BY
ALBERT NAPPER Esq, M R C S, L S A
FOUNDER OF THE SYSTEM, CRANLEIGH, SURREY

Six of its twenty-three pages are devoted to a lucid explanation of the need for village hospitals, and another four to details of the more serious of 100 listed patients. To appreciate the full impact of his creation on what was a fairly typical rural community we must look to the alternative facing the sick poor of Cranleigh before 1859. The nearest hospital was St Thomas', still conjoined at that time with Guy's near London Bridge. The patient with serious illness or injury had either to suffer in his own home, frequently little more than a hovel, over-crowded and ill-furnished, or to be carted (literally) thirty-five miles over poorly-made roads to London, a journey which many patients failed to survive. There was one other alternative, to be admitted to the workhouse and "nursed" by untrained hands. The choice could be little less agonising than the illness.

Napper recognised the impossibility of the village surgeon, however skilled, being able to offer adequate care under these conditions. "It appeared to me" he wrote,[7] "that it was only required to reduce the scale of the institution by establishing a hospital on a small and inexpensive plan, commensurate with the capabilities of the staff to secure ... the means of alleviating many of the evils and inconvenience so severely felt." "The Public", he continued, "appear to be labouring under the delusion that the majority of cases admitted into a hospital require, for their successful treatment, the united deliberations of a highly skilled medical and surgical staff, whereas, with an occasional rare exception, they may be equally well treated by any ordinarily well-qualified surgeon, aided by the advantages of good nursing, generous diet, and comfortable lodging." The building to be converted needed to be neither costly nor elegant, and big enough to house up to six patients, the number which he considered came within the scope of one nurse and helper. Should it be contemplated to *build* a hospital there was no better design, he felt, than that common to his part of Surrey, ie brick or stone walls for the ground floor, and timber, weather-tiled without, and lath and plaster within, for the upper part of the house. This cottagey type of building made the labourer feel at home. For many years architects tended to stress the cottage element to the detriment of the hospital.

You will have noticed that Napper used the term "village hospitals" in his title. This conforms with the first of three principles which, according to Horace Swete's *Handybook* were the basis of the "system" which he "founded". The third principle was that the cottage hospital should be open to all medical men who care to make use of it. It was Napper's second principle which was to cause the greatest controversy. It read:

> Equality of privilege to subscribers in recommending patients, the patient paying a certain sum, according to his means, weekly towards his maintenance.

Hitherto voluntary hospitals in county towns and elsewhere had, with few exceptions such as Dr Smith's Infirmary at Southam, made no charges to the patients, who were now, under Napper's rules, to contribute a sum which might be equivalent to half their weekly wage (five shillings a week was not unusual). This aspect of his "system" was given a general accolade, especially by a later writer, Henry Burdett, the great hospital administrator and historian, who was to call it the jewel in the crown of the cottage hospital movement. Meantime Napper himself charged no fees, an act which brought disapproval from the *British Medical Journal* which suspected (quite unjustifiably) that this was a devious way of achieving self-advertisement.

In the event the first 100 patients in Cranleigh Hospital contributed very little. As Napper himself pointed out "77 were parish paupers, who were virtually being attended by the respective medical officers gratuitously; 7 were persons totally without means of paying, and the remaining 16 were all in humble circumstances."

130 years later, looking back on Napper's three principles in the perspective of time, it is difficult to feel that they represented the major features of his "system", or that the cottage hospital movement would have foundered without them. Within a few years the bed-limit of six was frequently broken, charges for patients were levied or not levied according to local decisions and free access to all local practitioners, although generally welcomed was not always enforced. Yet the number of new foundations grew fast from 1864 onwards. By 1866 they were being recorded at the rate of one every four weeks, and by the end of the century over 300 had been counted, in Great Britain alone. The idea had been taken up in other parts of the world, especially New England where according to Henry Burdett some forty cottage hospitals sprang up in the last quarter of the century.

The cottage hospital movement undoubtedly began in Cranleigh under Albert Napper. Whether his was the first to be founded or not, or even whether it should compete for the title at all (being a village hospital according to his own writing) is of academic interest. I have not mentioned two tiny hospitals founded by Mr A A Davis, one in Fowey in 1859 and the other in nearby Par Consols in 1862. Mr Davis himself gave the credit for starting the movement to Napper. Nor have I so far included a dark horse which Horace Swete alludes to in the tail-end of the appendix to his book - a surgical hospital set up in 1842 (and perhaps earlier) in the village of Wellow near Nottingham where an enthusiastic surgeon named Mr Squire Ward included in his repertoire such operations as lithotomy, lithotrity, amputations at the thigh and shoulder, excisions of joints and removal of cataract, "all recovering", according to Mr Ward in a letter to Horace Swete, "without the use of carbolic".

By this time I am no longer able to count the number of Woozle-tracks that have appeared since I began to follow them, and no longer feel that it matters. What is important is the dynamic enthusiasm of the early pioneers, particularly Albert Napper of Cranleigh and Horace Swete of Wrington, who set up the highest of hospital care for the humblest members of the community, in a concept which has resisted all attempts at destruction to this day. It is difficult to think of any social institution which has so effectively brought together the members of a community in a common cause, outside war, over-riding all divisions of creed, race and social standing.

COTTAGE HOSPITAL DIETARY TABLES.

CRANLEIGH.

Ordinary Diet.—Meat (uncooked) ¾lb. daily ; butter ¼lb., tea, 2ozs. weekly. Bread and cheese *ad libitum.*

WRINGTON.

Ordinary Diet.—Meat ½lb., bread 1lb., potatoes 1lb., beer 1 pint, rice or arrowroot 2ozs. daily ; tea 3ozs., sugar ¼lb. weekly.

TEWKESBURY.

Ordinary Diet.—Meat 3lbs. (for males), and 2lbs. (for females), sugar ¼lb., butter 4 to 6ozs. weekly.

The ordinary diet for adults is subject to such alteration or modification as may be deemed advisable by the medical officer. With him also rests the power of ordering extras, as eggs, poultry, fish, jellies, wine, brandy, ale, or porter. *Sick Diet*, consisting of broth, tea, puddings, sago, arrowroot, milk, &c., is ordered as required by the medical attendant in each individual case.

10. Cottage Hospital Dietary Tables, 1870 from Horace Swete's Handybook of Cottage Hospitals

Before finishing there is just one medical man who must be mentioned and given the last word. He is Dr Spencer Thomson of Burton-on-Trent who wrote a letter to the *British Medical Journal* which was published on November 10th 1854 suggesting a way of alleviating the "evil of the sick poor being treated in their own over-crowded dwellings ... by having a sort of "Cottage Hospital" for every one, two, or more villages ... that is, a small house in which two or three separate rooms and beds should be devoted to the reception of the sick". Spencer Thomson never put his idea into practice. Had he done so, it might well be his name, rather than that of Albert Napper which we honour today as the founder of the cottage hospital movement.

REFERENCES

1. A.A.Milne, *Winnie-the-Pooh*. Methuen 1926. Page 3 of the 1971 reprint of the 1965 paperback edition.

2. John R. Guy, "Of the writing of hospital histories there is no end" *Bulletin of the History of Medicine,* 1985, *59,* 415-420.

3. Reginald Fisher, *Medical History.* 1963, 268-70

4. Horace Swete, *Handybook of Cottage Hospitals.* London 1870

5. Norman Moorsom, *N. Ormesby Hospital.* 1982

6. E.J. Dennison, *A Cottage Hospital Grows Up.* 1963

7. Albert Napper, *Village Hospitals.* London 2nd 1865 Edition

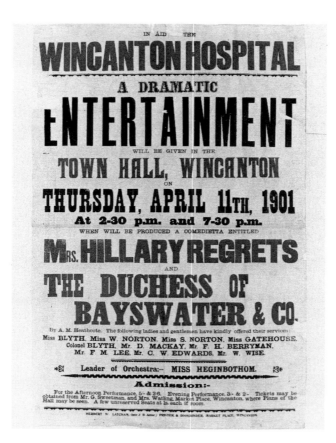

11. (left) Fund raising for a cottage hospital. Wincanton 1901 *(By courtesy of Eugene Taglione).*

12. (right) The Fever Van, by L S Lowry (1887 - 1976), painted in 1935. *(By courtesy of the Walker Art Gallery, Liverpool).*

THE SHADOW OF THE FEVER VAN

John R. Guy

L.S. Lowry is acknowledged to be one of the greatest British artists of the twentieth century. Finding his inspiration in and around Salford, Lowry determined to record for posterity scenes and impressions of the industrial landscape of provincial England. One of his canvases depicts a terraced street, peopled by men and women exhibiting in their posture and gaze a mixture of curiosity and apprehension. Their attention and ours is focussed upon a sinister, black-painted vehicle drawn up before the door of one of the houses. It is the isolation hospital ambulance awaiting its child patient, another victim of diphtheria or scarlet fever. Lowry entitled his painting *The Fever Van*. This paper will be concerned with differing perceptions of the role of the fever van; those of the medical officers of health, whose power it symbolised; those of the private medical practitioner, whose authority it sometimes undermined; and those of the patient's family and neighbours, to whom in some ways it was a threat.

There is no doubt that the powers of the medical officers of health, symbolised by the fever van, were resented by patients' families. How general or widespread that resentment was it is impossible to say, but there is evidence indicating both active and passive resistance to the desire of the MOHs to isolate scarlet fever sufferers.

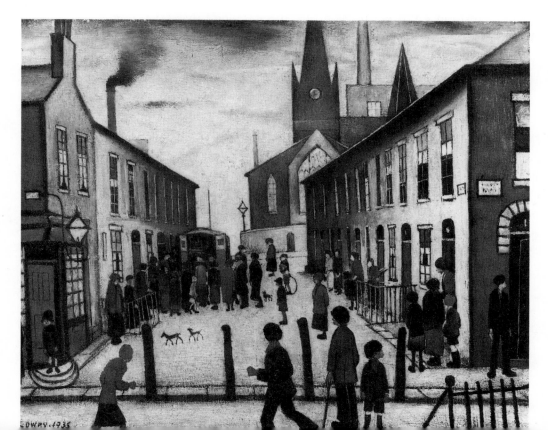

The necessity of obtaining a magistrate's order for the removal of a patient can be taken as evidence of active resistance. Such a case is recorded in the Register of the Truro Isolation Hospital in March 1907, when three children of one family, aged 9, 6 and 4 respectively, were admitted. As their admissions occurred on two successive days, the family must have put up a sustained resistance.[1] Few, perhaps, went to the lengths of a costermonger's wife in 1890 who, despite a magistrate's order refused to submit herself and her child, both suffering from scarlet fever, to hospital admission. She barricaded herself into her home, and even after the sanitary inspector and two policemen forced an entry had to be carried, still resisting, to the ambulance.[2]

Passive resistance took a variety of forms. Concealment of a case was always a temptation. Matthew Hay, MOH for Aberdeen, estimated in 1891 that of 84 cases dealt with in one month of an epidemic, 27% had not been attended by a doctor or notified, being "accidentally" discovered by his sanitary staff.[3] E.H. Snell, MOH for Coventry, believed that only about half the cases reached isolation hospitals,[4] and he was probably over-optimistic. Wynter Blyth, MOH for St Marylebone, reckoned that under a quarter - 24.8% - of scarlet fever cases were treated in hospital in 1892.[5] Even when allowance is made for the fact that many towns did not possess isolation facilities by 1892, that compulsory notification did not extend throughout England and Wales until 1899, and that some cases were isolated at home, it is hard to escape the conclusion that efforts were made by some families to conceal outbreaks. Such a temptation could be especially strong where livelihood was at stake. A diagnosed outbreak on a farm could result in a prohibition on the sale of dairy produce.

Passive resistance also took the form of a refusal to modify habits and routine. Henry May, President of the Birmingham and Midland Branch of the Society of Medical Officers of Health in 1889-90, was one who showed understanding of this problem, but parents were more often characterised as "careless", "thoughtless" or "wilful" by his colleagues. Desquamating children continued to play with their friends in the street[6] and to mix with neighbours.[7] Their parents expressed "annoyance" if the inspector endeavoured to curtail that freedom, especially if doing so interfered with their own avocation or social intercourse.[8]

Ignorance and fear underlay much of the resistance. However carefully the need for isolation was explained, the mechanics of the transmission of scarlet fever, only imperfectly understood by the doctors themselves, was well-nigh incomprehensible to many lay people. The MOH for Huddersfield, James Kaye, gave a telling example of this failure of understanding. He had found that children excluded from school because of an outbreak were nonetheless still being sent to Sunday School.[9] Parents not only failed to isolate their infectious children, but themselves continued in defiance of instructions to the contrary working in trades or occupations which brought them into direct contact with large numbers of other people. Dr Ridley Bailey of Bilston instanced a woman who continued to serve in her greengrocer's shop whilst nursing her child, and another who maintained her milk-round.[10] Such refusal to co-operate was punishable by law, as in the case of a Wolverhampton laundress who continued her business whilst her children had scarlet fever. She was found guilty of "wilful exposure", and fined 40/- plus costs, with a month's imprisonment if she defaulted.[11] Inevitably such action led to hostility towards the MOHs, and their inspectors, who were seen as "snoopers".

Ignorance was not confined to the artisan classes. James Kaye of Huddersfield castigated schoolteachers. He condemned the practice of sending healthy children to enquire after absent schoolmates, as not infrequently the "little enquirer" was asked into the house, and thus put at risk of infection. He also rounded on boarding schools for what he termed the "reprehensible habit" of disbanding pupils to their homes on the appearance of infectious disease, thus facilitating its spread from one community into others.[12] Schoolteachers, Kaye felt, should give sympathetic and intelligent co-operation to the MOH and his staff in combatting outbreaks. The implication of his remarks is that he was not receiving it.

Doctors and nurses themselves could be guilty of ignorance. In 1893 a nurse caring for the children of a High Wycombe brewer herself contracted scarlet fever. She was sent home to Woking by rail, travelling in a compartment with other passengers "although the rash was well out" and her temperature 101.8°. The arrangements had been made by the doctor attending the children.[13]

Such cases were cited by the MOHs to strengthen their calls for the extension of the 1889 Notification Act and for a greater provision of isolation hospital accommodation, focussing as they do on the inadequacy of domiciliary care. They nonetheless illustrate that there was a widespread misunderstanding of the nature and transmission of infection, and that that misunderstanding could give rise to resistance to the requirements of the MOH and his staff.

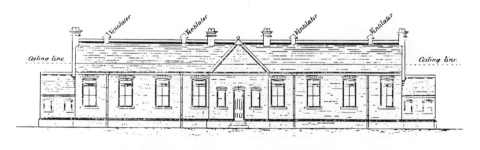

BOROUGH OF WARRINGTON
INFECTIOUS DISEASES HOSPITAL.

ELEVATION OF A TWELVE BED PAVILION.
SCALE 16 FEET TO AN INCH

Ths Longdin
Borough Surveyer.

13. An Isolation Hospital "pavilion", erected in accordance with a design (Model Plan C) published by Richard Thorne Thorne of the Local Government Board. 1888. Many similar blocks were built in the 1890's.

Fear goes hand-in-hand with ignorance. In the case of scarlet fever that fear arose in two clearly defined areas, one related to the home and the other to the hospital. Isolation was but one prong of a trident wielded by the MOH. The others were notification and disinfection.[14] Unfortunately disinfection could have a highly destructive effect, which at least in artisan households, was cause for fear and distress. H.J. Hutchens, Demonstrator of Bacteriology at the University of Durham College of Medicine in 1906, spelt out the process of disinfection in forthright terms. The child's books and toys were to be destroyed, its bedroom disinfected by the application of concentrated solutions of powerful germicides to the floor, bed, walls and furniture. Wallpaper was to be stripped and burned.[15] Hutchens was concerned with diphtheria, but similar measures were adopted for scarlet fever. The wholesale havoc and destruction that these procedures would cause is easily imagined, however necessary they might have been, but neither Hutchens nor others referring to disinfection seem to show any awareness of the resentment and heartbreak that might result. An exception was Henry May, who counselled his colleagues to be sensitive to the fact that their actions involved what he termed the invasion of the home.[16] More common was the attitude of Francis Fremantle, MOH for Hereford, who took parents to task for concealing clothes and toys from the disinfectors.[17] An added anxiety was that clothing, bedding and portable items were often removed with the little patient from the home to the isolation hospital, where the disinfecting apparatus was housed.[18] Child - or children - along with their intimate belongings, which in the case of poorer families may have been few, pathetic, cherished and obtained only after considerable sacrifice, were removed under distressing circumstances from the home. In such cases it is no exaggeration to say that the shadow of the fever van falling on the threshold could bring fear and anxiety.

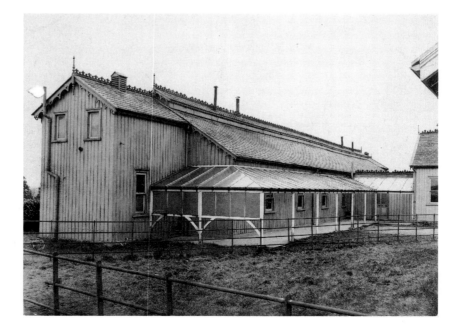

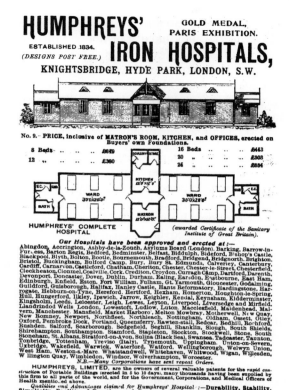

14. (right) Advertisement for Humphreys' Iron Hospitals, commonly used for isolation pavilions. No fewer than one hundred and seventy are listed as having been built in the British Isles and overseas. The advertisement appeared in The Medical Annual for 1902.

15. (left) A pavilion at the Bath Statutory Hospital, Claverton Down. The buildings were erected c1880 and demolished in 1933 when the hospital was rebuilt in stone. The later buildings were demolished in 1989, after final closure of the hospital.

There was also fear of the hospital itself. In most cases the buildings were sited some distance from the centres of population. Hidden behind high walls, fences or hedges, with limited access, the hospital had the air of what one former patient described succinctly as a "prison-camp".[19] At Truro in 1907 it was decided that relatives enquiring after patients could be admitted during one afternoon hour daily to the garden leading to the hospital entrance.[20] At Sherborne in Dorset convalescent patients, under supervision, in fair weather were permitted to stand in the yard and wave to relatives, themselves confined to the unmetalled lane outside of the gate.[21]

The behaviour of the patients in hospital was strictly regulated, and an authoritarian regime was itself a cause of resentment to those whose children had been accustomed from an early age to roam freely, playing in the streets, courts and yards. In 1892 the MOH for Nottingham, Dr Boobbyer, spoke of the necessity of keeping patients in bed for three weeks "whether they liked it or not".[22] In 1913 the authors of a paper on the outdoor treatment of scarlet fever could speak of their patients being "subjected" to that treatment[23] and record that all were forbidden at any time in cold weather to put their arms from under the bedclothes, to sit up or get up from the bed. They expected their "orders" to be carried out, and those who "from perverse notions" disobeyed, were wrapped and pinned into their blankets or sheets. The effects of this upon the minds of children - mostly aged 5 to 10 - already disoriented by sickness and removal from home, need no comment.

Overwhelmingly patients in isolation hospitals at this date came from the poorer classes of society. Small and overcrowded houses, sometimes occupied by two or more families, rendered home isolation for them next to impossible.[24] Although referring to Melbourne, Australia, Frank Scholes' verdict that not one private house in fifty could supply adequate facilities for home isolation also held good in Great Britain.[25] But many of the hospitals were badly designed and constructed and erected on waste land.[26] Wynter Blyth condemned some as having the appearance of cowsheds and being destitute of comfort.[27] In a revealing phrase he concluded that "only the poorest class under compulsion" could be induced to use them.[28]

This created a different fear, this time in the minds of middle or upper class families. Fear that their children would be isolated for six or seven weeks in open wards - glass cubicles were only gradually introduced[29] - with those of the working class. It is interesting to note that the MOHs themselves, when strongly advocating hospital isolation, made remarks like "would we not all gladly isolate our children *or at least our servants* in hospital?"[30] Macmartin Cameron, MOH for Wigtown, in a passionate defence of isolation hospitals,[31] called them "socialistic".[32] Some would not have regarded that description as laudatory. Where adequate isolation could be secured at home and the expense of a resident nurse incurred, then this was preferable. For Claude Rundle, Medical Superintendant of Fazakerly Hospital, Liverpool, "adequate" meant a large and well-ventilated room for the patient, the reservation of a "whole upper flat" for patient and nurse, and the rigid exclusion of all relatives.[33] The addresses of patients admitted to both the Truro and Taunton Isolation Hospitals in the years before World War I reveal a majority from working class backgrounds. The obvious exceptions are those of patients admitted from local institutions, at Truro nurses from the Royal Cornwall Infirmary[34] or students from the training colleges;[35] at Taunton from the boarding schools. In 1908 thirteen boys were admitted in little over a fortnight from Kings College;[36] in 1913 seventeen cases in October and November from Taunton School. What these patients had in common, regardless of age or sex, whether in Cornwall or Somerset, was that they were resident in institutions at a distance from their homes. For them there was no question of domiciliary care. There was no alternative to the isolation hospital.

The shadow of the fever van also fell upon the polished doorsteps of the private medical practitioners. Some doctors resented the need to notify the MOH of cases of specified infectious diseases. They saw it as an intrusion into their practice. When Edward Marriott of Nottingham called compulsory notification "un-English"[37] he was indirectly venting his spleen upon the MOHs and their inspectors. In the minds of some practitioners the salaried medical officers of health must have resurrected old prejudices against that other group of doctors who had accepted employment and lay management, the Poor Law medical officers. The Notification Acts of 1889 and 1899, which required the private practitioner to inform his salaried colleague of certain cases of illness, and then surrender that patient's management to him, cannot have been other than a bitter pill for some to swallow. Armand Trousseau, who had given the first clear clinical description of scarlet fever,[38] had spoken to his students of the "resignation so becoming in intelligent persons who feel for their absolute incompetence to judge medical questions ..."[39] That lay deference to the clinical omniscience of the private practitioner was threatened by the intrusive powers of the MOH and his lay staff. It is not therefore surprising that J.G. Blackman, MOH for Portsea Island, in 1892 counselled consultation between the MOH and the patient's medical attendant before that patient was admitted to hospital, if at all possible. He reminded his audience that the admission of a patient could mean "pecuniary loss to the medical attendant", and a private practitioner thus offended in his pocket might well be unco-operative over notification and isolation in the future.[40]

Such sensitivity was uncommon. The Public Health Act of 1875 had been a victory for those who advocated the isolation of fever patients in special hospitals. Among their most ardent advocates was Richard Thorne of the Local Government Board, whose report *On the use and influence of hospitals for infectious diseases*, published in 1882, dominated thinking on the subject for a quarter of a century. Thorne believed that the most useful function of such hospitals was to receive the initial cases of an infectious disease, and thus, by prompt isolation, prevent its further spread. Roger McNeill's famous book, *The Prevention of Epidemics & the Construction of & Management of Isolation Hospitals*, which appeared in 1894, with its utopian vision, was an almost inevitable development of Thorne's thesis, and Thorne himself was very much alive, his continuing advocacy of such hospitals assisting the great expansion in their numbers in the 1890s.[41]

Following his lead, emphasis was at first placed on the preventive role of isolation hospitals, but within a very few years that emphasis changed. In 1889 St Clair Shadwell had called isolation hospitals "a sure and safe method of preventing the spread of infectious diseases"[42] but in the very same year Henry May had warned that there was no "royal road" to prevention.[43] By 1892 MOHs such as Joseph Priestley of Leicester were seeing isolation hospitals not as a sure means of stamping out diseases such as scarlet fever, but "merely" as a way of controlling epidemics.[44] By 1898 the value of the hospitals themselves was being openly questioned.[45] In 1892 Rollo Russell had said that anyone could be a carrier of infection. Every case of sore throat in an infected house had the potential for transmitting scarlet fever.[46] With less than 50% of cases removed to hospital,[47] as a measure of preventive medicine, the isolation hospital had failed. Money would be better spent on inspectors, health visitors and teachers.[48]

Yet for many years the fever van continued to rumble through the streets, the wards were filled, the text-books advocated isolation.[49] But the hospitals' advocates had shifted their ground. Their provision was now seen as society's moral duty, to give patients the advantages of skilled nursing and "excellent medical treatment".[50] Although by the turn of the century outbreaks of the disease were usually mild, the mortality in the over-fives very low - perhaps less than measles - and complications rare, admission to hospital and isolation for six or seven weeks remained the norm. Having created the system, its authors felt the need to defend and justify it by using it to the full. The hospitals were undisputedly valuable for diphtheria and typhoid, but admissions for scarlet fever predominated until at least World War I. The hospitals were there, so they had to be used. They were used because they were there. But by 1900 at the latest, some MOHs had begun to realise that when it arrived at the gate, the shadow of the fever van fell across a white elephant.

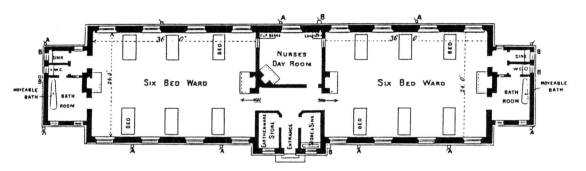

16. Plan of Pavilion. 1888. The 'moveable bath' could be brought into the ward and placed by a patient's bed.

REFERENCES

1.   Cornwall R.O. B/T 180. Truro Isolation Hospital Register of Patients 1897-1921. (not normally available for consultation under the "100 year rule".)

2.   *Public Health*, 1890-91, **3,** p 147

3.   ibid p 237

4.   E.H. Snell, The admission of infectious cases into General Hospitals. *Public Health*, 1898-99, **11,** pp 703-713, p 706

5.   Wynter Blyth, The isolation of the infectious sick in hospitals. *The Sanitary Record*, 30 October 1896, pp 378-382, p 378

6.   *Public Health*, 1891-2, **4**, p 7; Francis Wood & John R. Guy, *Well fenced in*: *The Forty Years of the Sherborne Isolation Hospital*. Forthcoming

7.   *Public Health*, 1889-90, **2**, p 508

8.   Dr Robertson (MOH St Helens), Compulsory isolation in certain infectious diseases. *Public Health*, 1892-93, **5**, pp 141-144, p 143

9.   James Kaye, The prevention of infectious diseases in schools. *Public Health*, 1893-94, **6**, pp 215-219, p 219

10.   *Public Health*, 1889-90, **2**, p 508

11.   ibid, 1891-92, **4,** p 7

12.   Kaye, art.cit

13.   *Public Health*, 1893-94, **6**, p 197

14.   J.Groves, On Isolation Hospitals. *Public Health*, 1892-93, **5**, pp 3-4, p 3

15.   H.J. Hutchens, Diphtheria: its prevention and treatment. *Public Health*, 1906, **18,** pp 337-356, p 351

16.   Henry May, The isolation of infectious diseases in hospitals. *Public Health*, 1889-90, **2**, 297-301, p 298

17.   Francis Fremantle, The value of isolation hospitals. *Public Health*, 1906, **19,** pp 1-22, p 6

18.   cf the advertisement for Washington Lyon's Patent Steam Disinfector, *Public Health,* 1889-90, **2**, opp p 112. Francis Wood & John R Guy, op cit

19.   Wood & Guy, op cit

20.   Cornwall R.O. B/T 180. 2 September 1907

21.   Wood & Guy, op cit

22. *Public Health*, 1892-93, **5,** p 137

23. H.M. Cargin & T.G. Shand, The outdoor treatment of scarlet fever. *Public Health,* 1913, **26**, pp 327-332, p 328

24. St Clair B. Shadwell, The need of infectious hospital accommodation for the suburban districts of the metropolis. *Public Health,* 1889-90, **2**, pp 266-67, Fremantle, art cit, p 5

25. F.V.G. Scholes, *Diphtheria, Measles, Scarlatina*, 2nd ed Melbourne, 1927, p 311

26. Robertson, art cit, p 143

27. Blyth, art cit, p 380

28. ibid

29. C. Killick Millard, The influence of hospital isolation in scarlet fever. *Public Health*, 1900-01, **13,** pp 462-503, discussion on pp 501-2

30. Sir Shirley Murphy, *Public Health*, 1906, **19,** pp 1, 13

31. Macmartin Cameron, Concerning the utility of isolation hospitals. *Public Health*, 1896-97, **9,** 224-226

32. ibid, p 225

33. Claude Rundle (ed), *Ker's Manual of Fevers*, OUP, 3rd ed 1927, 2nd impress 1932, p 99

34. Cornwall R.O. B/T 180, 30 April 1907

35. ibid 1 June 1906, 20 May 1909, 16 Sept 1910

36. Somerset R.O., Taunton Isolation Hospital Admissions Register 1904-1940, case nos 2527-2539 for Kings College; nos 2924, 2927-31, 2933, 2935, 2937, 2940, 2942-43, 2947-48, 2950-52 and 2956 for Taunton School. (Not normally available for consultation under the "100 year rule".)

37. *Sanitary Record*, 1900, **26,** p 124, quoted by John M. Eyler, Scarlet Fever and Confinement: the Edwardian debate over isolation hospitals. *Bulletin of the History of Medicine*, 1987, **61** no 1, pp 1-24, p 7. (Although the debate to which Eyler refers reached its climax in the early years of the 20th century, it had, in fact, got well under way in the 1890s, a point that he does not make clear.)

38. In 1861. See Armand Trousseau, *Lectures on Clinical Medicine delivered at the Hotel Dieu, Paris* trans from the 1868 edition by J.R. Cormack, vol 2, London, 1869, pp 161-211

39. ibid, p 199

40. J.G. Blackman, Some points in connection with the removal of patients to isolation hospitals. *Public Health*, 1892-93, **5,** p 4

41.   Eyler, art cit, p 2

42.   Shadwell, art cit, p 266

43.   May, art cit, p 298

44.   *Public Health*, 1892-93, **5** p 182

45.   Snell, art cit, p 706

46.   Hon Rollo Russell, *Epidemics, Plagues and Fevers: their causes and prevention*. London, 1892, pp 259, 260

47.   Edward Walford, The influence of hospital isolation upon scarlet fever in Cardiff. *Public Health*, 1903-04, **16,** pp 676-686, p 676

48.   H. Beale Collins, *Public Health*, 1906, **19,** 1, p 18

49.   eg Rundle, op cit, p 99

50.   Blyth, art cit, p 379

BATH, 1790.
CASUALTY HOSPITAL.

Directions for the RECOVERY *of the* APPARENTLY DEAD *by* DROWNING, *and the various kinds of* SUFFOCATION.

I. THE RESTORATION of HEAT is of the greateſt conſequence to the return of LIFE: when therefore the body is taken out of the water, the cloaths ſhould be ſtripped off; or, if naked at the time of the accident, it muſt be covered with two or three coats, or a blanket, or any thing anſwering the purpoſe that can be moſt eaſily procured. The body ſhould then be carefully conveyed to the neareſt houſe, with the head a little raiſed.—In *cold* and *damp* weather the unfortunate perſon ſhould be laid on a bed, &c. in a room that is moderately heated:—In *ſummer*, on a bed expoſed to the rays of the ſun, with the windows open, and not more than ſix perſons admitted; a greater number may retard the return of life. The body is to be well *dried* with warm cloaths, and gently rubbed with flannels, ſprinkled with rum, brandy, gin, or muſtard.—FOMENTATIONS of either of theſe ſpirits may be applied to the pit of the ſtomach with advantage.—A warming pan covered with flannel ſhould be lightly moved up and down the back; bladders, or bottles filled with hot water, heated bricks, or tiles wrapped up in flannel, ſhould be applied to the ſoles of the feet, palms of the hands, and other parts of the body.

II. RESPIRATION will be greatly promoted, by cloſing the mouth and one noſtril, while, with the pipe of a bellows, you blow into the other with ſufficient force to inflate the lungs; another perſon ſhould then preſs the cheſt gently with his hands, ſo as to expel the air: thus the natural breathing will be imitated. If the pipe be too large for the noſtrils, the air may be blown in at the mouth. Blowing the breath can only be recommended when bellows cannot be procured.

III. THE BOWELS ſhould be very ſoon inflated with the *fumes of Tobacco*, and repeated three or four times within the firſt hour; but if circumſtances prevent the uſe of this vapour, then CLYSTERS of this herb, or other *acrid infuſions with ſalt*, may be thrown up with advantage.——The FUMIGATING MACHINE is ſo much improved as to be of the higheſt importance to the Public; and if employed in every inſtance of apparent death, it would reſtore the lives of many of our fellow creatures, as it now anſwers the important purpoſes of *fumigation, inſpiration,* and *expiration.*

IV. AGITATION has proved a powerful auxiliary to the other means of recovery: one or more of the Aſſiſtants ſhould therefore take hold of the legs and arms, particularly of boys, and ſhake their bodies for five or ſix minutes; this may be repeated ſeveral times within the firſt hour. When the body is wiped perfectly dry, it ſhould be placed in bed between two healthy perſons, and the friction chiefly directed, in this caſe, to the left ſide, where it will be moſt likely to excite the motion of the heart.

V. When theſe Methods have been employed for an hour, if any brewhouſe, bakehouſe, or glaſshouſe, be near, where *warm grains, aſhes, lees,* &c. can be procured, the body ſhould be placed in any of theſe moderated to a degree of heat very little exceeding that of a perſon in health. If the warm bath can be conveniently obtained, it may be advantageouſly uſed in conjunction with the earlieſt modes of treatment.

VI. ELECTRICITY ſhould be very ſoon employed, as it will increaſe the beneficial effects of the other means of recovery on the ſyſtem. "The ELECTRICAL SHOCK," ſays Mr. KITE in his *Eſſay* on the *Recovery* of the *apparently dead,* " is to be admitted as the teſt or diſcriminating " characteriſtic of any remains of animal life; and ſo long as that produces *contractions,* may the " perſon be ſaid to be in a *recoverable* ſtate; but when that effect has ceaſed, there can no doubt re- " main of the party being abſolutely and poſitively dead."

VII. If ſighing, gaſping, convulſions, or other ſigns of returning life appear, a tea ſpoonful or two of warm water may be put into the mouth; and if the power of ſwallowing be returned, a little warn wine or brandy and water may be advantageouſly given. When this gradual approach towards recovery is obſerved, and breathing and ſenſibility returned, let the perſon be put into a warm bed, and if diſpoſed to ſleep, as is generally the caſe, give no diſturbance, and he will awake, after a ſhort time, almoſt perfectly recovered.

The above methods are to be uſed with vigor for three or four hours; for it is a vulgar and dangerous opinion to ſuppoſe perſons are irrecoverable, becauſe life does not ſoon make its appearance; an opinion that has conſigned an immenſe number, of the ſeemingly dead, to the grave, who might have been RESTORED TO LIFE by *reſolution* and *perſeverance.*

17. Instructions for resuscitation of the apparently drowned. Bath Casualty Hospital.

A PIONEER ACCIDENT SERVICE: Bath Casualty Hospital, 1788-1826

John Kirkup

Not only did 1988 witness the 250th anniversary of the Bath General Hospital, the first hospital to specialise in rheumatic diseases, but also the 200th anniversary of the opening of the Bath Casualty Hospital, perhaps the first hospital designated to receive accident victims only.

The Trustees' Minute Book of the Casualty Hospital[1] dated 1st January, 1788 states:

> Whereas, since the great Increase of Bath, frequent complaints have been made of the Want of an Hospital or Place for the Reception of Day Labourers and other poor Persons meeting with sudden Accidents. We, whose Names are hereunto set, having opened a Subscription for providing a House, (to be called the Casualty Hospital), a Nurse, Medicines, and all other Necessaries, for receiving such poor Persons as shall meet with sudden Accidents in the Parish of Walcot; (that Parish having engaged to pay the Sum of five shillings per Week for every Person meeting with such sudden Accidents, during his or her continuance in the said Hospital). And when all or any of the Parishes of St Peter and St Paul, St James and St Michael in the City of Bath, shall agree to the like Conditions, they also shall be allowed the Benefit of this Institution. And We hereby associate ourselves as Trustees for the above Purpose and agree to the following Rules and Orders for the Management of the said Hospital.

> Signed, J.Sibley, S.Griffith, G.Ramsay,
> T.Neate, W.Anderdon.

Rule 3 stated:

> Daniel Lysons MD and Mr James Norman, Surgeon, having humanely offered to attend the Patients of this Hospital Gratis, resolved that their offer be thankfully accepted and that they be respectively appointed Physician and Surgeon to the same.

Rule 4 stated:

> At meetings, Physician and Surgeon can give opinion, but not vote.

Rule 7 stated:

> Mary Davies hired as Nurse, weekly salary 4/- when no patients, 6/- for one, 8/- for two and then 5/- extra per week per additional patients for maintenance and washing.

On 3rd January, 1788, the Minute Book noted, "At a meeting of the Trustees this Day resolved that Miss Somerville's House in Kings Mead Street (Illustration 18) be taken at a rent of Twenty Guineas a year, for one Year ... as a Hospital". Fortunately this building has survived.

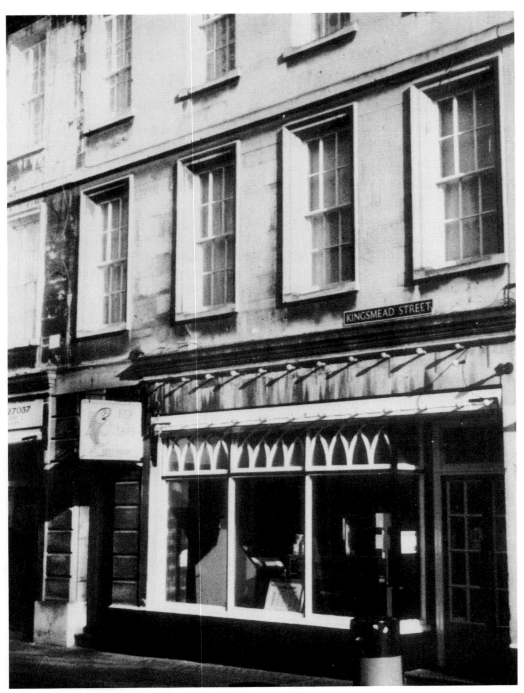

18. Miss Summerville's House in Kingsmead Street, Bath.

And on 7the January, 1788, the *Bath Journal* reported:

> We have the satisfaction to inform the Public that a Casualty Hospital for the Reception of Sudden Accidents is opened in Kings Mead Street ... Subscriptions and Benefactions are received by the Treasurer William Anderdon Esq at the Bath and Somersetshire Bank, Milsom Street.

Despite these accounts, it is probable that the surgeon James Norman played an important role in establishing the Casualty Hospital. Trained in Bristol, he was on the staff of both St Peter's Hospital and the Bristol Royal Infirmary until his sudden unexplained resignation when he moved to Bath in 1783. Munro Smith in his *History of the Bristol Royal Infirmary* writes:

> James Norman was of rough exterior and blunt, unpolished manners, and was not fitted to succeed in a place like Bath. He was, nevertheless, a sound practitioner and good operating surgeon. I believe he was the first on the Infirmary Staff to amputate at the shoulder joint ... the patient recovered perfectly.

Arriving in Bath without a hospital appointment and finding practice highly competitive, he must have backed the idea of the Casualty Hospital at an early stage to ensure his election as surgeon *gratis*. Nevertheless, within two years of this appointment he requested a gratuity and the Trustees gave him £42, " ... on account of his extraordinary trouble."

With the opening of the Casualty Hospital, we can identify three categories of injured patient in Bath: the destitute, unemployed inmates of the workhouse, alone entitled to use its infirmary, the rich and well-to-do who could pay for surgical attention in their own homes, and the employed poor whose crowded, unhygienic homes were inadequate for home care, even if surgeons' fees could be paid, but who were now entitled to use the Casualty Hospital.

A unique feature of this institution was its enlightened policy of no financial barrier for admission of the injured, provided their accident took place in Walcot parish. As we shall see, this geographical limit was never strictly applied and soon patients came from all areas of the city and outside. In general, admission to hospitals in Britain at this time depended on the possession of a subscriber's ticket and hence some personal relationship with a subscriber, which must have effectively denied help to many. By contrast, free access to the Casualty Hospital was a pioneering departure.

Patients and Hospital Statistics

Unfortunately, the only details concerning patients are to be found in the local newspapers, the *Bath Journal* and the *Bath Chronicle*. Their reports are somewhat sporadic and obviously incomplete, yet nevertheless strongly supportive of the hospital for the first five years or so. Thereafter reports become extremely infrequent. Here are examples of the early accounts.

The *Journal* of 25th February, 1788 states:

> Admitted into the Casualty Hospital last week - Martha Godsell, with a contused wound in her foot - Geo Jefferis and Charles Finch, much contused in their bodies by falling in of the quarry at Lansdown Place - Isaac Mills with a fractured leg - ALSO RELIEVED, John Gibson whose thigh was contused by a waggon going over it.

The 2nd June, 1788 issue states:

> Richard Grenfell about 13 years met stone carts in Bathwick Lane and his leg broke. Samuel Hathaway, about 14 years, slipping from a bank, a cart ran over his legs resulting in a violent bruise on one of his ankles. John Baker, postillion, standing at the head of his horses in Bath Easton, the horse took fright, beat him down and fractured his skull. Benjamin Sykes, a plumber, fell from a window in Peter Street by which he was dangerously bruised. The above 4 persons were all admitted into the Casualty Hospital.

It is noteworthy that Bathwick Lane and Bath Easton are outside Walcot Parish.

The *Bath Chronicle* records some of the above patients but also others not published in the *Journal*. For example, on 13th November 1788:

> Admitted to the Casualty Hospital last week. John Morgan with an incised wound of the leg; John French, contused thigh by a fall from a scaffold; and John Davis, with a fractured skull from the kick of a horse.

And on 4th March 1790:

> John Neate a lad about 15 years of age, fell from the top of one of the buildings in the New Square, by which accident he broke his arm and was otherwise much bruised. He was immediately taken to the Casualty Hospital, where he is now in a fair way of recovery.

And on 22nd April 1790:

> Thomas Wilson (a boy about 14) fell from the scaffold of one of the new buildings in Bathwick Fields, by which accident he fractured his leg, his arm and one of his thighs, and was otherwise much bruised. He was immediately taken to the Casualty Hospital, where he expired next morning.

The number of young boys admitted in their early teens is a significant; no doubt they were inexperienced and perhaps rash in clambering over scaffolding and exposing themselves to other risks. Here are further reports from the *Chronicle*. On 22nd July 1790:

> ... John Davis, a lad of 14, being at work in one of the new houses in Bathwick, a bucket laden with stones falling with great violence ... struck him so violently on the head, and though instantly taken up and carried to the Casualty Hospital, he did not survive many minutes.

On 21st October 1790:

> Admitted into the Casualty Hospital George Date, a lad about 16, with a violent contusion of his back and loins, by a fall upwards of 40 feet from the gutter of a house in Lansdown Place.

The Trustees' Minute Book mentions the printing of 600 copies of the *Annual State of the Hospital* at the end of 1788 which were to be sent, one to every subscriber, although the list published in the newspapers only totalled 136 subscribers. For 1790, 800 copies were to be printed and sent to every subscriber, coffee house, library and the Public Rooms. Curiously this printed document is not mentioned after 1798 when only 300 copies were printed. Happily the newspapers re-printed the details of those for 1789 to 1792 inclusive, for none of the original documents appear to have survived, whilst the newspaper reports for 1790, 1791 and 1792 are analysed into groups for diagnosis. Other figures were published in the annual *Bath Guides* of the period but the same statistics were repeated over several years and cannot be considered reliable. The collected evidence concerning in-patient admissions, discharges, deaths and out-patient attendances from 1788 to 1796 is shown (Fig 1). The work-load increased steadily from the beginning to 1792 when all reliable information ceased; the figures for 1794 and 1796 suggest a considerable decline in activity but as these are extracted from the *Bath Guides*, they may not be accurate. Evidence from the Trustees' Minute Book in January, 1791 reported the ordering of two extra bedsteads as " ... all beds in the house amounting to ten having been filled ..."[1] and thereafter it is known the hospital enlarged to a maximum of fifteen beds before its final

	1788	1789	1790	1791	1792	1794	1796
Admitted	45	50	76	102	105	68	66
Discharged well	37	43	69	91	100	-	-
Died	6	3	6	7	2	-	-
Out-patients	-	254	413	600	888	572	419

Fig. 1: BATH CASUALTY HOSPITAL - Patient statistics for 1788 - 92, 1794 and 1796.

closure. Almost from its opening, there was a fund established for a larger hospital and as early as June, 1788 the Pauper Charity for medical care in the city made approaches to pool their resources for the construction of a joint hospital. By January, 1820 matters were coming to a head and the trustees minuted, "... premises inadequate ... must devise plan for purchasing or building" and later that month, "As no 4, Pierrepont Street for sale at 1,000 guineas - resolved that Mr Norman to purchase it forthwith."[2] The sale however fell through and with great reluctance the trustees finally agreed to a merger with the Pauper Charity, which had become the Bath City Infirmary in 1792. This junction finally took place in 1826 when their union became the Bath United Hospital, now the Royal United Hospital.

The diagnostic analyses for out-patients treated in 1790, 1791 and 1792 show remarkably few fractures and dislocations whilst almost 50% of the total consists of contusions. In the days before X-ray examination, it is probable a proportion of the contusions were actually fractures. The newspaper case reports suggest that the majority of the burns and scalds involved small children. In 1792, the separate category of "abscess" is noted. This confirms a deliberate policy of the trustees in March that year, to accept responsibility for surgical cases other than accident victims when they minuted, "... that two beds ... be kept for chirurgical cases ... or any other case in surgery which requires confinement".[1] However less than two months later they reported that:

... the great and rapid increase of buildings prevents an extension of the Charity beyond Casualties and a fear that Parishes for many miles around will take advantage.

Nevertheless as the in-patient analysis of 1792 shows (Fig 2), two patients were admitted with an abscess and two for the "greater operation", that is lithotomy for bladder stone. Thus the policy to widen the surgical base of the hospital persisted and later included surgical tuberculosis, as reported in the *Chronicle* for 2nd January, 1794 when admission

	1790	1791	1792	%
Fractures	21	18	22	} 23.5
Dislocations	1	1	2	
Contusions	39	52	41	47.8
Lacerations	8	28	30	23.9
Scalds and burns	6	3	4	4.7
Abscesses	-	-	2	-
Greater operation	-	-	2	-

Fig 2: BATH CASUALTY HOSPITAL In-Patient diagnoses for 1790 - 92.

was given to, "… Joanna Richards, a white swelling in her knee, whose leg being amputated, is in a fair way of recovery." It is noteworthy that fractures and dislocations accounted for almost a quarter of admissions as opposed to 2.6% of out-patients.

None of these figures demonstrated the challenge posed by drowning in the near-by river Avon. The newspapers record a steady stream of unfortunates, taken out of the river and then transported to the Casualty Hospital where the means recommended by the Humane Society to restore the apparently drowned usually proved ineffective, principally due to delay in getting them out of the river. On 19th May, 1818 a complaint was made:

… by Captain Fane respecting the conduct of Servants of this Hospital in regard to the case of a man lately brought in drowned. Resolved that the Matron and Nurse acted culpably… in deciding case beyond reach of medical assistance …[2]

Nonetheless prolonged efforts do appear to have been made to resuscitate these cases and, as early as 1790, an instructional leaflet under the name of the Casualty Hospital was published discussing mouth to mouth ventilation, tobacco smoke enemas and electrical shock, among other measures recommended.

Conclusion

There is little doubt the Bath Casualty Hospital was successful in helping accident victims, many of whom were injured during the building boom in the city of the late eighteenth century. Initially serving the parish of Walcot, it later accommodated accidents sustained throughout the city and adjacent country-side. The standard of surgical care appears to have been excellent, firstly under the experienced James Norman until he retired in 1816 and secondly under his son George Norman, later senior surgeon at the United Hospital.

The author has searched for evidence of similar institutions in the eighteenth century without success and the next earliest hospital specifically designed for the injured appears to be the Poplar Hospital for Accidents, opened in 1855 to receive cases from the adjacent London docks. It ultimately became a general hospital and was finally closed in 1974.[3] The construction of the Manchester Ship Canal involved large numbers of workmen and accidents were anticipated with the provision of three hospitals along its length; these were active from 1887-1893 under the control of a Surgeon-Superintendent, Robert Jones, the well-known orthopaedic surgeon.[4] Lorenz Bohler, who founded the Vienna Accident Hospital in 1925, mentions in his book[5] an earlier establishment at Graz, and the Birmingham Accident Hospital opened in 1941, continues to restrict admission to injured victims.

Even if the Bath Casualty Hospital is not the first of its kind, it surely deserves recognition as a pioneering venture in responding to the needs of the injured and in offering help without financial barriers. It can be claimed a provincial medical success and, after 200 years, it would be appropriate to commemorate the story with a plaque at 38, Kingsmead Street - which currently is rated a good class fish and chip shop.

REFERENCES

1.   Bath Casualty Hospital. Minutes of Trustees monthly meetings, 1788-1817. Wellcome Manuscript 1094

2.   Bath Casualty Hospital. Minutes of Trustees monthly meetings, 1817-1826. Wellcome Manuscript 1095

3.   Lloyd, C.J. (Personal communication), 1988

4.   Seddon, H.J. The Manchester ship canal and the colonial frontier. *Journal Bone & Joint Surgery*,1961 **43** *B*: pp 425-433

5.   Bohler, L. *The Treatment of Fractures*, translated by E. Hey Groves. Bristol, 1935

UROLOGICAL CIRCLES

Clive Charlton

The evolution of the flexible urethral catheter corresponds with the period during which rubber was introduced into Europe, and used for its manufacture. Urological circles, the title of this paper, has at least two interpretations. One refers to the shape into which a catheter can be adapted as a result of incorporating rubber in its making so that it can be bent into a circular shape and thereby accommodated into a gentleman's hat. Another interpretation refers to the cyclical nature of history, whereby we have recently readopted a practice (namely intermittent self-catheterisation) which had been abandoned earlier in the century for a supposed improvement.

Prior to the age of rubber, rigid tubes of tin, copper, bronze, silver or gold were passed along the urethra, and in Roman times clay catheters were also used. Through the centuries, hollow stems of onions, rushes and other plants have also enjoyed their popularity, but my story begins with a thesis written in 1699 by Dr Grubeling of Helmstadt,[1] who starts by giving an account of the history of the catheter. This thesis is one of a collection made by Albrecht Von Haller, published in five volumes in the mid-eighteenth century, under the title of *Selected Surgical Disputations*. These theses or essays were subjects suggested by a professor, and so the candidate wrote an essay with supporting and contrary arguments which he had to present in public in the presence of the professor, and such members of the university who cared to attend. Haller preserved these essays on account of the full and accurate description of a disease, of new instruments invented or of unusual precautions adopted. The fourth volume deals with stone, lithotomy and the disease of joints. They are printed in Latin, and usually begin with an invocation to God or a dedication to the professor. The subject of the thesis is stated briefly with the etymology of the surgical terms used, introducing when possible some indication that the candidate knew a little Greek, even if it were no more than the Greek characters.

The collector of these essays, von Haller,[2] was a remarkable man, and probably the greatest bibliographer we have known, classifying fifty-two thousand publications of a botanical, surgical, medical and anatomical nature. He was also a physiologist engaged in the research of muscle and nerve irritability and made a study of the intercostal muscles. This polymath, in addition to being a non-operating surgeon, was a professor of anatomy, physiology and botany for seventeen years at Göttingen (a town between Frankfurt and Hanover), and a poet. His best known work was that on the Alps, which went into twenty-two editions. His other activities included declining the Chair of Botany at Oxford, being elected a Fellow of the Royal Society and entertaining Casanova at his home. His *curriculum vitae* was further augmented by being the author of 13,000 scientific papers. In 1752 he was made a Baron of the Holy Roman Empire by Emperor Francis I.

To revert to the flexible catheter, Avicenna, the Prince of physicians, who lived at the end of the first millenium, used animal skins, stuck together with cheese glue to form what must surely be one of the earliest disposable flexible catheters. A rather more durable flexible catheter of spiral silver was invented by the Dutch surgeon, Cornelius Solingen in 1706 and is to be found in the collection of the Royal College of Surgeons at Lincoln's Inn Fields.

Another polymath who was busy designing a similar flexible catheter for his brother, was Benjamin Franklin, who between reading a paper to the Royal Society on electricity in 1752, and being a signatory of the Declaration of Independence, was exercising his mind in the direction of a flexible silver catheter.[3]

The breakthrough in the development of the flexible catheter came with the use of rubber. Although Columbus, on his second voyage to the New World, had observed the Indians in Haiti, using balls "made of the gum of a tree", the serious business of discovering a chemical process whereby the crude mass of cake of rubber could be made pliable and malleable had to wait until the mid-eighteenth century when resin or caoutchouc was brought over from Quito in Ecuador to Paris in 1736. The physicians Herissant and Macquer[4] (a grandson of Scottish folk who left their homeland to escape religious persecution and went to live in Paris, he acquired an MD, and later became one of the greatest of French chemists) introduced pure ether as a solvent, and they were able to mould the rubber and make surgical instruments. The first elastic gum catheter is credited to Monsieur Bernard (a jeweller and goldsmith) who in 1779 covered the silk or twisted goat hair (forming the basic framework of the catheter) with elastic gum. In the two-volume treatise written by Monsieur Desault,[5] the Principal Surgeon to the Hotel Dieu, this invention of a flexible, smooth, pliant and firm catheter is described as "One of the most fortunate discoveries that has enriched the art of surgery this present century". A few years later, a medical student at Edinburgh, James Syme, discovered a solvent for India-rubber. This latter appellation came about since Europeans started using rubber obtained from the East Indies, to rub out pencil marks. In 1818, Syme wrote a letter to the *Annals of Philosophy*,[6] describing how he distilled from coal tar a fluid named Naphtha, in which he immersed slips from the cake of caoutchouc. This swelled to form a homogeneous mass which was moulded into a suitable shape and dried on exposure to air.

Syme's name is still associated with the operation of amputation of the foot, by transection of the tibia and fibula at the level of the malleoli. Like so many Scots surgeons, he made his way to London, was appointed to staff of University College Hospital, but was not particularly happy there, and soon resigned that post to return to Scotland. Similarly his son-in-law left Glasgow for King's College Hospital, but there he stayed to achieve fame and ennoblement as Lord Lister. Syme's discovery was patented in 1823 by the Scottish chemist Charles Mackintosh. He placed a solution of naphtha and rubber between two layers of fabric, and so avoided the sticky and brittle surfaces that had been common in earlier single-textured garments treated with rubber. The double-textured waterproof cloaks henceforth became known as mackintoshes.

However the effect of warming by the body resulted in the rubber catheter becoming soft. Further progress was halted until Goodyear in the USA invented the process of vulcanization in 1839. He added lead and sulphur to the rubber, which imparted a durable quality not hitherto possessed.

Soon after this, Auguste Nelaton, a well known Parisian surgeon and physician to Napoleon III, had the first catheter of vulcanized rubber made.[8] This was improved upon, and patented for commercial use by James Archibald Jacques, the works manager of a rubber factory in England. Some of us still remember being offered a Nelaton or Jacques catheter by the theatre staff for urological procedures, and it was with these catheters that the Victorians were taught to pass this instrument upon themselves. To facilitate the introduction of the catheter, Auguste Mercier[9] recommended the incorporation of an elbow bend or coudé near the tip, and later Jean Louis Petit introduced a further improvement; the double elbow or bi-coudé catheter.

Everard Home, a son-in-law of John Hunter, was one of the first surgeons in this country to encourage patients to catheterise themselves. He instructed them in this art, and recommended that the catheter should not be passed more frequently than six-hourly. So we come to the period of intermittent self catheterisation. In the USA, the "ten cent catheter"[10] came into vogue and we learn of one such catheter being used 1,200 times. In the UK, a patient catheterised himself 35,000 times[11] (or four times a day for 24 years).

The art of catheterisation requires considerable skill, and in the last quarter of the nineteenth century one of its most noted exponents was George Buckston Browne.[12] He describes being summoned from London to Paris, to relieve a rich American of urinary retention, the local surgeons having failed in their endeavours. His fee for crossing the channel and successfully undertaking this manoeuvre was 500 guineas! It is of interest that George Buckston Browne failed his MB, and qualified by passing the conjoint examination. He also failed his FRCS, and consequently never had a hospital appointment, but in 1874 he was taken on as a private assistant by Sir Henry Thompson, the doyen of urological surgeons in England, for the sum of £200 per year. He bought himself a house in Wimpole Street, where he lived for the rest of his professional life, being released after 1pm of his duties as an assistant, and began to build up his own practice. He had in his consulting rooms a stall, in which the patient would stand, whilst Buckston Browne sat on a stool facing the adversary and so passed the catheter with great expertise and gentleness.

He obviously acquired a considerable reputation, and he further describes another fairly lengthy journey from London to Anglesey, to deal with an MP who was also a director of the Midland Railway. Once again, the local surgeons had failed to pass a catheter, and B.B. with his deft touch succeeded. However, having battled his way home, he was recalled three days later, since the catheter had fallen out. This time he insisted that a special train be laid on for the return journey, accompanied by his patient. The MP was installed in one of Buckston Browne's numerous nursing homes, which he owned in the vicinity of Wimpole Street, making it possible to care for his patients on foot, since he never learned how to drive a motor car. Buckston Browne described the articles needed by a patient who was to catheterise himself for the rest of his life. He suggested a cardboard box about the size of a shoe box, wherein were contained seven catheters each positioned in its own compartment for each day of the week. The catheter lubricant was a pot of vaseline with ten per cent of oil of eucalyptus. In addition, there was a glass tube which was to be held upright in a wooden stand, into which four to five ounces of a fresh mercurial solution prepared by dissolving a pellet of perchloride of mercury in boiled water was added, and used to sterilize the catheters. All these were to be placed in a large tin box, useful for travelling, or if going on a shorter trip, then two catheters and the lubricant were placed in a metal pocket case which was attached by a ring and chain to the belt round the patient's waist. This latter was essential if the catheter was not to be lost, as happened to one fellow who was clambering over Snowdon. He lost it between some rocks. Browne described how many well known patients who led public lives and were successful as singers and artists, could manage this regime for up to 39 years. Furthermore, they became so adept at this manoeuvre that one of his actor friends could pass his catheter under a rug in a crowded third-class carriage, and another performed the acrobatic feat seated upon his saddle.

The surgical fraternity paid B.B. the compliment of having him elected honorary FRCS. This honour he repaid in full, by buying Charles Darwin's old home, Down House, in Kent, and donating it to the College for the purposes of surgical research. His generosity and wealth were such that he spent £100,000 in renovating and equipping this building. So the Buckston Browne Research Farm came into being, which remains active to this day, despite the attentions of the anti-vivisectionists. These activities were recognised by a knighthood.

The next stage in the development in the use of the catheter was a self retaining catheter. The object of this was to avoid the inconvenience of it falling out, and so the necessity of repeated catheterisation, with its attendant complications, one of which is that of perforating the urethral wall with the catheter, which then runs parallel to the natural channel and establishes a false passage. More commonly, a relatively minor abrasion of the urethra heals with scar tissue and results in a narrowing of the channel, known as a stricture. As a result there is considerable difficulty in passing a subsequent catheter down the pinhole-sized lumen of the urethral tunnel.

One of the first catheters designed for long-term retention was invented in 1853 by the French surgeon Reybard.[13] He devised a balloon made of either rubber or gold beater's skin, made of the caecum of pigs or sheep, which was inflated with water or air through a channel running the length of the lumen of the rubber catheter. A somewhat less sophisticated measure for retaining a catheter *in situ*, was that adopted by Sir Henry Thompson (George Buckston Browne's tutor and guide) who anchored tapes to the pubic hairs. Contrary to first impressions, he was in fact a cultured man, some of his own art works being hung in the Royal Academy. He was also an enthusiastic collector of blue and white Nanking porcelain and was married to a celebrated pianist. He was a most hospitable man, and his dinner parties were famous and traditional in that the number of guests (all male) was limited to eight. They were held at 8 o'clock and there were eight courses. These octaves were held on each Thursday evening that he was in town and on the three hundredth occasion the Prince of Wales was an honoured guest.

This versatile Victorian,[14] as his biographer Zachary Cope called him, reached the apogee of his career by successfully treating Queen Victoria's uncle, Leopold, the King of the Belgians, for bladder stones, where other famed Europeans had failed. His reward was a knighthood at the age of 47. Being securely established in practice, he went on to devote his energies to a number of varying enterprises. In 1874, he was a founder member and elected president of the Cremation Society of England, pioneering against considerable opposition this method of the disposal of the dead. He then successfully turned his attention to the matter of getting museums and galleries in London to open their doors to the public on Sundays, and this he did through the agency of the Sunday Society. His baronetcy in 1899 is partially attributed to his generous gift two years previously to the Royal Observatory at Greenwich, of a large photographic telescope manufactured for him in Dublin. His final fling, when aged 80, was his devotion and passion for the motor car, which led him to write a booklet on the care and maintenance of these vehicles.

Self retaining urethral catheters gave way to self retaining suprapubic indiarubber catheters. The senior surgeon at the Westminster Hospital, Mr Barnard Holt, described in *The Lancet* in 1870[15] a rubber catheter with wings, which opened in the bladder and kept it *in situ*. Some two months later, there is a letter written to *The Lancet*, from his home in Saville Row, stating that as a result of the overwhelming demand for his catheter, supplies were temporarily exhausted; but that Mr Baker of 244 High Holborn, was making some more which would be available in two weeks time. This concept of the self-retaining catheter was further advanced some twenty years later when de Pezzer[16] gave an account of his mushroom-ended catheter, rapidly followed by one designed by Malecot,[17] with a wing-tipped end for its retention. These are still in use today.

Reverting to self-retaining urethral catheters, Tuchmann,[18] of Moorgate Street, on the north side of the city of London, described an ingenious double catheter. An outer 19 FG silk webb coudé catheter with an eye at the convexity of the elbow, was passed into the bladder; this was followed by a 10FG straight catheter down the lumen of the coudé catheter. The advancing end of the inner catheter passed through the eye at the coudé and protruded for an inch into the bladder. The two open ends of the catheter were then tied together. This he described in the *BMJ* in 1893. Many prototypes of balloon inflating catheters were made, and it was not until 1933 that a catheter was commercially produced in Portland, Oregon, under the guidance of Hobart Dean Belknap.[19] It was assembled from parts made in the USA and France, and based on the principles of Reybard's first balloon catheter of 80 years previously.

During the 1930's , we again go the *full circle*, with respect to the treatment of rubber. When it is collected from the tree, it oozes through cuts made in the bark as latex. In the eighteenth and nineteenth centuries, the Indians and other workers then smoked this gooey material so as to give it a firm consistency, which was transported in a solid form, known as caoutchouc. I have described the difficulties encountered in getting these cakes of rubber back into a form which permitted it to be moulded, and later the development of vulcanisation to make it durable. In the early twentieth century, it became possible to collect this latex direct into drums, seal it and transport it across the world. As a result, it became possible to form rubber articles by dipping and coagulating the latex over metal rods, and so create a catheter and balloon in one piece, known as the integral catheter. It is then baked in an oven, which is the equivalent of the curing by smoking over a fire as undertaken by the Amazonian Indians. The first integral catheter with the balloon channel incorporated into the wall of the catheter was demonstrated by Frederick Foley,[20] to his colleagues at the American Urological Association Meeting in San Francisco in 1935. Since then we have seen the introduction of polymers and plastics for all types of catheter, but perhaps somewhat surprisingly, the use of the long-term self-retaining catheter is being questioned, and the final *volte face* is our enthusiasm for the Buckston Browne approach, namely, intermittent self catheterisation. Once again the industry has responded to our needs, and we now have a catheter, which on contact with fluid, has such a low coefficient of friction, that Sir George Buckston Browne's eucalyptalised white vaseline has become redundant.

I believe that we will soon complete another circle, by relaxing what has been an obsession, namely the belief that only sterile catheters can be passed with safety, and will revert to a more sensible and practical approach to what should be a domestic activity.

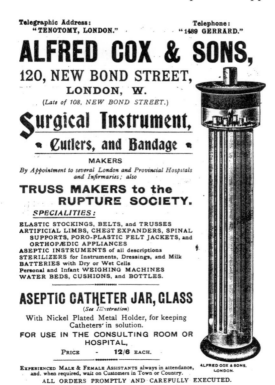

19.   Advertisement for an Aseptic Catheter Jar from The Medical Annual for 1902.

REFERENCES

1.   Grubeling, F C, *Dissertatio Medico-Chirurgica de Catheterismo*. 1699. In *Disputationes Chirurgicae Selectae*. Ed Albertus Hallerus, Laussannae 1760

2.   Power, D'Arcy, Albert von Haller and the Disputationes Chirurgicae Selectae. In *Proc of Vth Congress of the Internat Soc History of Medicine* (1925). Geneve Imprimerie Albert Kundig. 1926

3.   Pepper W, *The medical side of Benjamin Franklin*, p 28. Philadelphia, USA. 1911

4.   Herrisant, M and Macquer, P J, 1766. Observation Chimique in *Hist Acad Roy de Sc*. Année MDCCLXIII, p 49

5.   Desault, P J, *Parisian Chirurgical Journal*, **1**, 1794 p 163. Transl by Robert Gosling, London. Printed Bossey and Cheesewright, London

6.   Syme J, Letter written to *Annals of Philosophy*. 1818, **12**, p 112

7.   Goodyear, Charles, Improvement in the mode of preparing caoutchouc with sulphur for the manufacture of various articles. US Patent 1090. Filed by Nathaniel Hayward. Granted 24.2.1839

8.   Castiglioni, A, *A history of medicine*, p 715. Alfred A Knoff, NY. 1947

9.   Mercier L A, Memoire sur les sondes elastiques et particulièrement sur les sondes coudées et bicoudées. *Gaz Med de Paris*, 1863. 3rd series **18**: pp 365-7

10. Gouley, J W S, Notes on American Catheters and Bougies *New York Med J*, 1893 **58**:85

11. Murphy, L J T, *The History of Urology*, p 388. Charles C Thomas, Springfield, Illinois, USA. 1972

12. Dobson, J and Wakeley, C, *Sir George Buckston Browne*. Livingstone Ltd (Edin and Lond). 1957

13. Reybard, J F, *Traité pratique des rétrécissements du canal de l'uretre*. Labe, Paris. 1853

14. Cope, Z, *The Versatile Victorian*. Harvey and Blythe Ltd, London. 1951

15. Holt, B, A new form of catheter for retention in the bladder, *Lancet* 1870 i:p 261

16. de Pezzer, Nouvelles sondes urethrales et vesicales en caoutchouc pur très flexibles. *Cong Francais de Chir*, 1890 **5**:675-81

17. Malecot, A, Sonde se fixaut d'elle-même à demeure dans la vessie. *Arch de Tocologie et de Gynecologie*, 1892 **19**:321-3

18. Tuchmann, M, A new self retaining catheter. *Br Med J*, 1893 ii:pp 898-899

19. Belknap, H D, A new prostatic catheter bag. *Urol Cutan Rev*, 1933 **37**:pp 555-556

20. Foley, F E B, A self retaining bag catheter for use as indwelling catheter for constant drainage. *J Urol*, 1937 **38**:pp 140-3

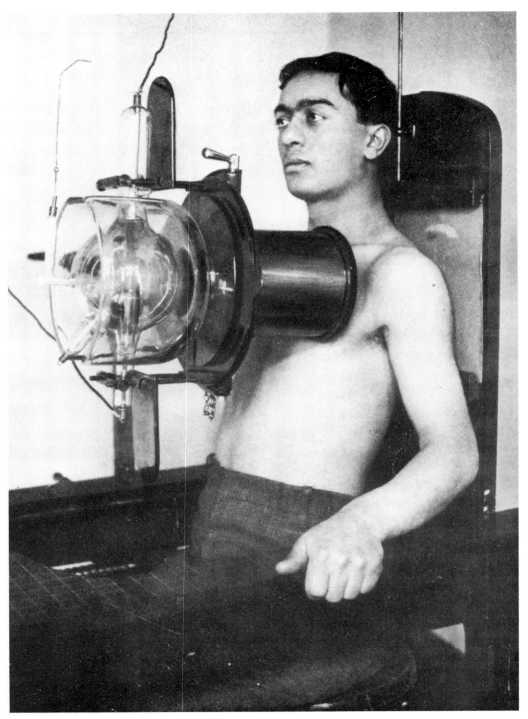

20. Radiography of the left shoulder in 1910. The apparatus is complex and cumbersome, and the uninsulated wires are carrying a potential of at least 50,000 volts.

FLYING SPARKS - Personalities in early South Western Radiology

Jean Guy

Radiology as a diagnostic technique began in February 1896[1], less than two months after the date of Röntgen's discovery of X-rays. The spread of this technique was phenomenally rapid. However radiology as a full time medical speciality, with a few notable exceptions in the major cities, did not develop until after the First World War and in some areas until after the second.

The larger hospitals of the South West of England acquired X-ray apparatus between 1896 and 1911, the pioneers being Cheltenham, Gloucester and Bristol General Hospitals, and Bristol Royal Infirmary. There was usually a medical officer in charge of the department whose activity in it, at least in the early years, was inversely proportional to his professional standing. Thus a general practitioner in a cottage hospital who had an interest in electrical gadgetry would probably operate the equipment and develop the films himself, whereas in a teaching hospital one of the surgeons or physicians would be nominally in charge, but the day to day work was often delegated to the house surgeon, out-patient sister or dispenser.

This arrangement was inevitable given the honorary nature of hospital appointments. Whether general practitioner or specialist, the doctor would derive his income from practice outside the hospital. Within the hospital his work might be regular and sometimes even onerous, but was never full time. The arrangement worked reasonably well for medicine and surgery. For various reasons it was not successful in radiology, and the demands of the speciality could lead to intraprofessional conflict.

To be successful, diagnostic radiology requires expensive equipment, operational expertise and experience in interpretation. Specialists in other medical fields have had difficulty in appreciating these facts. In the hospital records of the South West I have discovered in the committee minutes two examples of dispute arising from the management of the radiology services. One instance was in the Royal United Hospital in Bath, the other in the Royal Devon and Exeter Hospital, both during the First World War. The problem in Bath related to the purchase of apparatus, and in Exeter to the staff allowed to operate it.

During this period the X-ray apparatus in the Royal United Hospital was under the supervision of Dr George Edward Bowker. Born in Herefordshire in 1869,[2] he was educated at Edinburgh University, qualifying in 1891. Subsequently he was in private practice in Bath. By 1917, when the dispute took place, he was Senior Assistant Physician at the RUH. The establishment of the X-ray room in 1901 had been carried out by Bowker's predecessor Dr Preston King.[3] After a few years, he had the assistance of a nurse.[4] The emphasis in this department was on X-ray therapy rather than diagnosis.[5] By 1905 King's department was so busy that he resigned his post of Assistant Physician, retaining charge of the electrical department.[6] Bowker took practical charge at about the time of its re-equipping in 1911,[7] though King was still nominally head of the department.[8]

Bowker's name features in the minutes in relation to three important episodes. He was engaged in a prolonged controversy concerning the treatment of school children for ringworm, the commonest application for X-ray treatment during this period. The matter was resolved by the hospital making a charge of "3/- per sitting, covering cash and depreciation" but Bowker had to make his own arrangements with the Education Committee, from whom he asked half a guinea per sitting. This arrangement maintained the principle that the medical staff held honorary appointments.[9]

In 1913 the house committee received a letter from him drawing attention to the lack of X-ray tubes for the radiographic department.[10] The activities of an X-ray department of that time required several tubes, some for treatment and some for diagnosis. Bowker was referred to the "senior officer of the department", probably King, so that the request could be made to the medical board. Four years later the problem of X-ray tubes appeared again. He wrote to the management committee thus:

> Yesterday I learnt from Mr Sheppard that your committee only reluctantly agreed to the purchase of two new X-ray tubes for use in the electrical department. I was more than surprised to hear this and can only attribute this to lack of knowledge on the part of your committee of what such a department really requires to be able to work efficiently.
>
> My position as *Assistant Physician to the Electrical Department* has never been what I was given to understand it would be and has become quite unsatisfactory from my point of view. I therefore think my better course is to tender to your committee my resignation of that position forthwith as I cannot do justice to myself or the institution under present arrangements.[11]

Perhaps, now rising 48 years old, he was feeling frustrated in his hopes of a full honorary appointment to the hospital. If Bowker had expected to have his resignation rejected he was certainly disappointed. Matron was "asked to make arrangements for a nurse to attend the War Hospital for instruction in X-ray work"[12] and Bowker was not replaced at the Royal United Hospital by another doctor until 1921.[13]

Some X-ray equipment had existed in the Royal Devon and Exeter Hospital since 1898.[14] This was renewed three years later[15] and an Electrical Department set up in 1907.[16] Mr John Delpratt Harris had been in charge of this department since 1908, already qualified for 36 years and the senior surgeon at the hospital since 1896.[17] By the First World War he had been at various times president of the South West branch of the BMA, treasurer of the Devon and Exeter Medico-Chirurgical Society, MOH and JP of the city of Exeter and consulting surgeon of the lying-in charity; a man of great substance. His surgical papers were numerous, relating to such diverse topics as intracranial haematoma, pulmonary tuberculosis and goitre. From 1904 Harris undertook to train nurses in electrical work and massage and published a training handbook.[18] He also established from the outset that fees were payable for his services in the hospital by private patients. The medical officer was to receive two-thirds of the fee, the hospital one third.[19]

As in Bath, the emphasis in the Electrical Department was on treatment. The new installation of 1907 included "an electric immersion bath, ultraviolet light, high frequency apparatus, a four cell Schnee bath, ionic medication, Finsen Light and X-ray treatment."[20] In that year 21 X-ray photographs were obtained for the purpose of diagnosis and the X-ray apparatus in the casualty department was used 450 times, probably for screening or fluoroscopy. The workload increased apace, demanding several new tubes in 1910 and an "honorary photographer" or assistant medical officer in 1912.[21] By 1917 285 cases were photographed and 54 screened in the Electrical Department, referred to as the "Medical and Massage Department" in the Annual Report of that year. In casualty a further 113 cases were photographed and 98 screened.[22]

Almost every year requests for new or replacement apparatus appear in the committee minutes and are granted.[23] These included the storage batteries which Harris preferred to mains electricity for his equipment, a transformer coil, a fluorescent screen, a tube box and several tubes. The Electrical Department was regarded as sufficiently important to justify the setting up of an Electrical Subcommittee of the General Committee of the hospital, which dealt with many of the day to day problems of the department.[24]

In 1915 Harris resigned as senior surgeon to the Royal Devon and Exeter Hospital having reached the age limit, probably sixty-five years, but wished to continue as Honorary Medical Officer in charge of the Electrical Department "for at least another three years." At the end of that period he again requested renewal of his appointment "for not more than two years" which would take him to the age of seventy.[25] These renewals were granted without comment and probably with some thankfulness in view of the shortage caused by young doctors away serving in the war, including Harris's medical assistant Roper.[26]

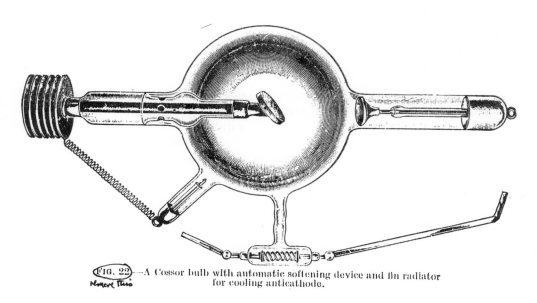

FIG. 22 —A Cossor bulb with automatic softening device and fin radiator for cooling anticathode.

21. An Xray tube of 1917 demonstrating special appendages for cooling the anticathode and controlling the vacuum in the tube.

During August 1918 a violent argument broke out during a meeting of the honorary medical staff. The minutes, if any existed, have not survived, but subsequent correspondence suggests the following course of events. The 1907 rules of the Electrical Department[27] specified that the house surgeon was permitted to operate the movable X-ray apparatus in the Casualty Department which was frequently needed for emergency work. In that month the house surgeon was seen to be using the X-ray tubes belonging to the Electrical Department, in defiance of the rules, which specified that these were reserved for the use of the Medical Officer in Charge. Sister Coy, the sister in charge, reported this to Harris, and was in turn reported to the medical staff. Harris upheld his nursing sister's action, having to explain by letter at some length the reason for his support and for the existence of the rules themselves.[28]

The tubes, he said, were not damaged but this was not the point at issue. Further explanation is as necessary for a modern audience as it was for Harris's colleagues. The tubes he is referring to, subsequently called "gas tubes", were not of a very high vacuum, Passing a current through the tube caused the gas within it to be absorbed by the glass of the tube. This increased the vacuum and made the current harder to pass, increasing the voltage required, and increasing the energy of the X-rays while reducing the quantity of radiation, to the point where no current would pass until the voltage was so high that the thin glass of the tube melted.

A low vacuum tube produced "soft" rays of low energy, often used to treat skin disease such as ringworm because they did not penetrate more than a few millimetres of skin. A high vacuum tube produced "hard" rays of high energy needed for radiography of thick body parts such as the pelvis. Any well run department had a wide range of tubes varying from very hard to very soft, and the tubes were changed around as their hardness varied from day to day. A "hard" tube became softer if rested for a few days, or after being gently heated, or by adjusting one of the ancillary projections of the tube.[29]

As Harris said:

> At present it is impossible for the makers of these tubes to guarantee the "quality" of a tube, nor whether a "hard" tube will become "soft" or a "soft" tube "hard". In view of this and as these tubes change their quality by use, it is very necessary that the Sister in charge should know the quality and characteristics of each tube so that she can select one suitable for the case under treatment. Excessive or injudicious use can ruin a tube, and if these tubes are to be used for casualty cases my work will be greatly embarrassed, for I could not then depend on the "quality" of any tube.[30]

Harris maintained the right of his departmental sister to enforce the rules of the department in his absence and to report any breach to him. This was an essential point, for he was not obliged under those rules to attend more than twice a week. He possessed his own X-ray apparatus and probably continued to act as an operating surgeon until he reached retiring age.[31]

Herein lay a source of conflict which was not resolved even when he retired, for his successor and former partner D Miller Muir would also have had honorary status. Frank Roper the assistant medical officer in charge of the department returned from the war in

1919, but by the next year was promoted to honorary physician.[32] There is evidence that from 1916 "photographic work", usually at this time meaning part or all of the process of radiography, was performed both by the dispenser and the dispenser's assistant. "For an extra £10 per annum and the assistance of an additional capable nurse" Sister Coy herself was persuaded to take on these duties, thus becoming one of the growing number of lay radiographers who appeared after the First World War.[33] In this way the day to day and the emergency radiographic work were delegated from medical to non-medical personnel in many hospitals.

GLASS CONTROL (CONSOLIDATED) ORDER, 1917.

Orders for X-Ray Tubes must be certified by the

Ministry of Munitions of War,
Optical and Glassware Supply,
22-23, Hertford Street,
London, W.1.

Customers wishing to order Tubes can either send their orders in duplicate direct to the Ministry for certification, or send us a post-card stating the Tubes which are required, and we will send a form which customers can fill up, and upon its return to us we will submit the order for certification to the Ministry.

22. An advertisement carried in a Watson & Son catalogue of c1917 - 18 indicating regulation of Xray tube supply during the First World War.

These examples naturally raise the question of whether there was similar intraprofessional conflict elsewhere and why similar problems arose in these two different hospitals at more or less the same time. A moment's consideration will reveal that this type of squabble is unlikely to be recorded in a hospital's annual report, in published articles in medical journals, or in obituaries. A thorough search has failed to reveal any other examples in the south west. So far as I am aware a parallel study has not been performed in other areas, either for radiologists or for other specialities. Historians of individual hospitals have used such archives, but are often strangely silent about the black spots within them. I should be very interested to hear of similar discoveries in other parts of Britain.

The dating of the conflicts is probably not a coincidence. There were two major shortages in the radiological practice of the First World War, skilled manpower and suitable glass for X-ray tubes. The departure of doctors to the front reduced the medical staffing inside and outside the hospitals, placing the burden of extra civilian work on those doctors remaining at home, in addition to the care of the sick and wounded sent home to "Blighty".[34] I have no doubt this added to the stresses and strains on the radiologists as well as their colleagues. The surviving departmental statistics in many other hospitals than Exeter tell a tale of considerably increased workload wherever there were staff available to perform the work. Roper's absence from Exeter on military service left an elderly and probably crotchety man in charge who had many other commitments. A rack of unused X-ray tubes waiting for the twice weekly consultant visit must have seemed a wicked waste to the house surgeon when his own were breaking down.

The shortage of X-ray tubes was a national problem. It would have made radiologists jealous of those good tubes which they possessed, as replacements were difficult to come by.[35] The price rose, of course, and this is the likely reason for the reluctance of the hospital committee in Bath to buy two more, though this was not made explicit. Although there were British glassmakers at this time, their numbers and their output had been much reduced by foreign competition and they were unable to produce the special soda-glass required for X-ray tube manufacture. The normal source of this was Germany. Before the end of the war British chemists had produced a practical formula for its production, and small-scale manufacture was occurring at home. Meanwhile American tubes and glass were imported.[36]

The problem of variable output from gas tubes was solved by technological improvements developed by Coolidge and the General Electric Company of America. The hot cathode tube was more reliable and its output could be varied at will. But its high cost and the conservative outlook of British radiologists ensured that it did not achieve universal acceptance in Britain for about fifteen years after its invention.[37] Paying for X-ray equipment remains a problem today.

To summarise, I have described two examples of conflict between early radiologists and their clinical colleagues. They arose for several reasons, explicit and implicit. Fellow-doctors on the hospital committees were unable to understand how X-ray equipment worked, and were therefore unsympathetic when additional or replacement equipment was asked for. They were also unaware of the difficulties inherent in operating this equipment. The problems were compounded and precipitated by wartime crises.

REFERENCES

The following abbreviations are used:

RUH   Royal United Hospital, Bath, Minute Books. These volumes are in the Royal Hospital for Rheumatic Diseases, Upper Borough Walls, Bath

EGCMB   Royal Devon and Exeter Hospital, General Committee Minute Book

EAS   Royal Devon and Exeter Hospital, Annual Statements

EESC   Royal Devon and Exeter Hospital, Electrical Subcommittee Minute Book

        The documents relating to Exeter are in the Devon Record Office, Exeter with an index number 1260F.

1.   E H Burrows, *Pioneers and Early Years, a History of British Radiology*. Colophon Ltd, St Anne, Alderney, C I, 1987, pp 35-41

2.   *Medical Who's Who* (1915) and *Medical Directory* (1896, 1901, 1916, 1919)

3.   RUH, **15** (1897-1902), p 364, 3 Jan 1901; ibid **16** (1902-1906), p 119, 4 May 1903; p 166, 2 Nov 1903

4.   ibid **16** p 214, 18 April 1904; p 216, 2 May 1904

5.   ibid **16** p 216, 2 May 1904; p 322, 3 April 1905

6.   ibid **16** p 365, 16 Oct 1905

7.   ibid **17** (1906-1913), p 324, 12 June 1911; p 341, 4 Sept 1911

8.   *Medical Directory* 1916

9.   RUH **18** (1914-1921) pp 236-7, 25 April 1917; p 238, 2 May 1917; p 239, 14 May 1917; p 241, 21 May 1917; p 244, 11 June 1917; pp 256-7, 3 Sept 1917; p 259, 24 Sept 1917

10.   ibid **17** p 441, 3 Feb 1913

11.   ibid **18** pp 262-3, 11 Oct 1917, letter from Bowker to committee

12.   ibid **18** p 265, 29 Oct 1917

13.   ibid **18** p 284, newspaper cutting of Annual Report for 1921

14.   These can be seen on display in the Postgraduate Centre, Royal Devon and Exeter Hospital, Barrack Road, Exeter. See also EGCMB HM 39, 2 Dec 1897

15.   EAS HA5, 1901

16.   ibid HA6, 1906, 1907 p 6; EGCMB HM41, 29 Nov 1906, 13 June 1907, 27 June 1907

17.   EAS HA7, 1908; EGCMB HM41 3 Sept 1908

18.   *Medical Directory* 1896, 1906, 1919, 1922, etc. The booklet's title is "Short Dict. of Electrical Treatm"; I have not been able to trace it or identify it more closely.

19.   "Copy of Resolutions suggested by the Medical Staff and Adopted by the General Committee, Wednesday 17 July 1907" (typescript filed in EGCMB HM41). EESC HM84, 17 July 1907

20.   EAS HA6 1907

21.   ibid HA7 1910; HA8 1912

22.   ibid HA10 1917

23.   eg EGCMB HM41, 3 Jan 1907

24.   Set up Tuesday 26 July 1904

25.   EGCMB HM42, 3 June 1915; HM43, 4 July 1917

26.   EAS HA10, 1919; EESC HM85, 28 Aug 1918

27.   EESC HM84, 17 July 1907

28.   EGCMB HM43, 15 Aug 1918; 19 Sept 1918; 26 Sept 1918; 10 Oct 1918; letters filed with EESC HM85 (i) from Harris to Cole dated 13 Aug 1918 (ii) letter from Harris to Electrical Subcommittee filed under 12 Sept 1918 (iii) letter filed under 7 Oct 1918

29.   David Walsh, *The Röntgen Rays in Medical Work*, London, 3rd edn, 1902, pp 43-45

30.   In 1922 Harris and D Miller Muir who succeeded him as Medical Officer in Charge of the X-ray, Radium and Electrical Department at the Royal Devon and Exeter Hospital were sharing an address at 45 Southernhay, Exeter, presumably Harris's private practice rather than his home. The date implies that he continued in that practice after retiring from the hospital. *Besley's Street Directory of Exeter, 1922*

32.   EAS HA11, 1920. Harris's immediate successor was J W Hodgson of Exmouth, already in his sixties, who was replaced by Muir in 1922

33.   EGCMB HM43, 15 May 1919

34.   Brian Abel-Smith, *The Hospitals, 1800-1948*, London, 1964, pp 262-3

35.   Permission to purchase tubes had to be obtained through the Ministry of Munitions of War (*Glass Control [Consolidated] Order 1917*)

36.   H J Powell, *Glass Making in England* (Cambridge 1923) pp 167-8, 172; Anon [Cuthbert Andrews Ltd] "Even for a man who ..." *RAD* June 1987, p 26; A K Smith-Shand, Radiology and Physico-Therapeutics, *J Royal Naval Medical Services* (1920) **6** pp 156-200 esp 167-174

      The problem was foreseen: Weir and Haldane in the House of Commons, as reported in *J Röntgen Society*, 1907, p 78

37.   Leonard S Reich, *The Making of American Industrial Research*, Cambridge, 1985 pp 88-91, 93

TO MEND A BONE: A Short History of the Management of Fractures

John Tricker

Fractures have occurred since the beginning of recorded time. They may be either closed when the skin has not been broken or open when the skin has been damaged and there is direct entry from the environment to the fracture site. The principles of the management of fractures are to reduce the fracture fragments to an anatomical position and to hold that position until the fracture has united; these were known to the ancient Egyptians.

Elliott Smith in 1908 reported the results of the Hearst expedition to the Nubian Desert. Here he found examples of splints which were used for holding reduced fractures dating from approximately BC 2600. These earliest known splints are now in the Museum of the Medical School in Cairo and in one of them is displayed the remains of a girl of approximately fourteen with an open fracture of the mid shaft of the femur, which had not shown any new bone or callus formation and was held with strips of wood, secured with linen bandages. These, however, not only immobilised the fracture fragments but also the knee joint as well.

Hippocrates in his second book describes methods of reductions of fractures using the scamnum and notes "that by such machines and such powers it appears to me that we need never fail in reducing any dislocation of the joint." After reduction Hippocrates applied the palms of his hands to adjust the fractured parts which were then bound up. Reduction was always in extension.

Galen used glossoconium which was a method of traction and counter traction, and it is his methods and those of Hippocrates which were used over the next 1000 years.

In 1314 Henri de Mondeville was writing a four part treatise on medicine. His fourth part was to cover fractures, dislocations and affections of bones. He began the introduction to this part "I cannot live long being asthmatic, consumptive, coughing and phthisical". He then unfortunately died which was an inauspicious start to the renaissance of the management of fractures.

Guy de Chauliac in 1363 appreciated the need of a knowledge of anatomy and also realised that callus was engendered with the help of God. He recognised that there were four parts in the management of fractures:

1.   reduction

2.   preservation of the equalised bone

3.   that the fracture needed to be bound with callus

4.   that the complications required remedy

He also was the first person to suggest the use of "a cord hanging over the bed or some other object for the patient to catch and help himself when he wishes to go to stool, to

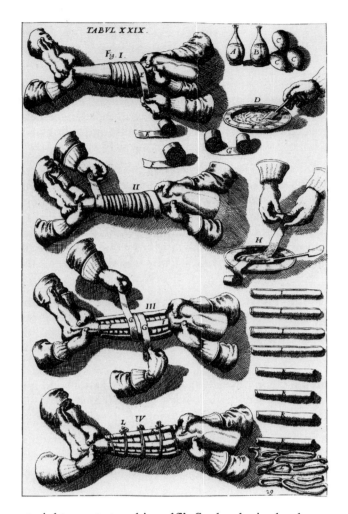

23. Bandage fixation of fracture of tibia *(from Scultetus Armamentarium Chirugicum. 1653).*

straighten or to turn himself". Such a device has been used since that time and the modern counterpart of such a cord is known as a monkey pole.

He not only realised that fractures could be reduced by traction, but also recognised the use of maintaining the reduction by balanced traction using the body weight as counter traction. "I attached to the foot a leaden weight passing the cord on a little pulley. It will keep the leg to its proper length". It is a very similar device that we use today in balanced traction.

Ambrose Paré (1510-1590) who made many metal artificial prostheses, deals with fractures in his Book XV. He devised an apparatus for the reduction of fractures and dislocations using ropes with traction and counter traction. He recognised the problems of diagnosing fractures and dislocations especially around the hips. He also recognised the positions of displacement of fracture fragments especially in fracture dislocations of the ankle joint.

In 1517, Gersdorf, a *Wundartz*, or bone setter, devised a splint which bears his name and which consisted of slats of wood bound together with thongs. These were then twisted and held with toggles through which a piece of metal was passed in order to stop the toggle untwisting and the thongs becoming looser.

Benjamin Gooch, who was the founder of the Norfolk and Norwich Hospital, devised a splint which is very similar to that of Gersdorf. The Gooch splint has continued in use until the present day.

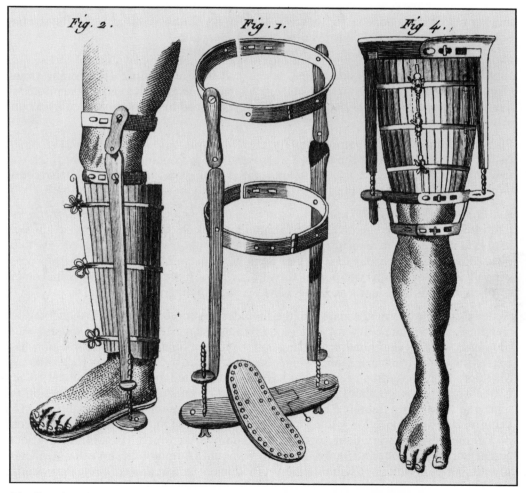

24. Gooch splint. *(from Benjamin Bell's "A Complete System of Surgery' 1791).*

John Hunter started the treatment of fractures on a scientific basis and Albrecht von Haller (1708-1777), a Swiss physician who held the chair in the University of Göttingen, experimented on the formation of bone and was the first to use the term *osteogenesis* in 1763. At that stage it was thought that bone was a substance deposited by the blood within the periosteum. Percival Pott (1714-87), who sustained an open fracture of his tibia, had an unusual treatment at that time in that he would not allow the limb to be amputated. Instead he rested it for an adequate length of time until the fracture and the skin healed. He later wrote his paper on fracture dislocations which was published in London in 1768. He felt strongly about the management of fractures and wrote: "The most inexpert and least instructed practitioner deems himself qualified to fulfil the part of the physician. He regards bone setting as no matter of science but as a thing that the most ignorant farrier may receive from his father and family as a kind of heritage". At this time Mrs Sarah Mapp was a popular bone setter. She lived in Epsom and her only qualification for the role was that her father was a bone setter. It was noted that her skill was insignificant but she had boldness, enthusiasm and considerable strength.

Other methods of maintaining the reduced fractures until union had taken place required substances such as waxes and resins, which had been used since Hippocratic times. Cheselden made plasters from linen and egg white, and in 1749 he used such a plaster on a boy with an open fracture of the humerus who had had his fracture treated by a bone setter.

Plaster-of-Paris was first mentioned by Eton in 1743 in his *A survey of the Turkish Empire*. In 1828 in Berlin, Deffenbach poured plaster into a box containing the limb which was known as a *platre coulé*. Mathijsen, a Dutch military surgeon, in 1854 used a coarse cotton cloth and finely powdered plaster.

Astley Cooper (1768-1841) in his *A Treatise on dislocations and fractures of the joints*, published in 1822 and regarded as the first modern book on the subject, says that "medical men find it so much easier a task to speculate than to observe, and they are too apt to be pleased with some sweeping conjecture which saves the trouble of observing the process of nature". Astley Cooper was putting forward scientific theories towards the management of fractures and this is not surprising as he was a pupil of John Hunter.

Astley Cooper treated a dislocation of the shoulder in a very similar way to that described and illustrated by Paré 200 years previously. He also suggested that certain splints should be hinged which makes him the forerunner of the idea of functional or cast bracing which is used today and which has more recently been advocated by Sarmiento in Italy, although Sir James Paget has often been said to have first suggested the use of functional braces. Lister with his new methods for the management of infection made an impact on the management of open fractures, but it was Malgaigne who pioneered external fixation by using a claw-like device for holding a transverse fracture of the patella. Towards the end of the nineteenth century there was a major controversy, which has continued to some extent into the twentieth century, about the amount of immobilisation that a fracture should have. Lucas Championnière conducted a strenuous campaign stating "immobilisation caused severe damage producing muscle wasting, and stiffness of joints". This became known in the 1930's as the fracture disease.

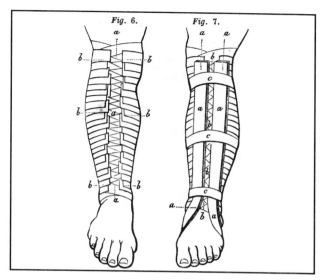

25. (left) Mathijsen's plaster-of-Paris bandage for fracture of tibia. 1854.

26.. (below) Joseph Amesbury's splint. 1831.

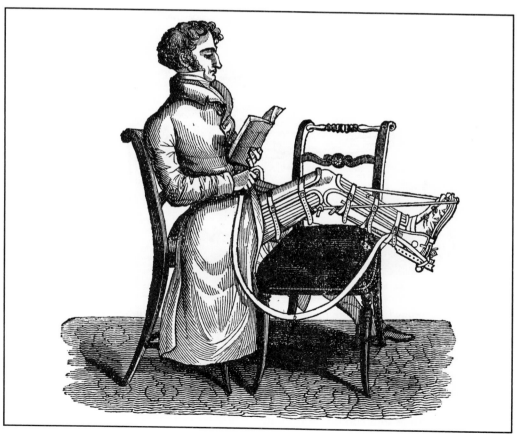

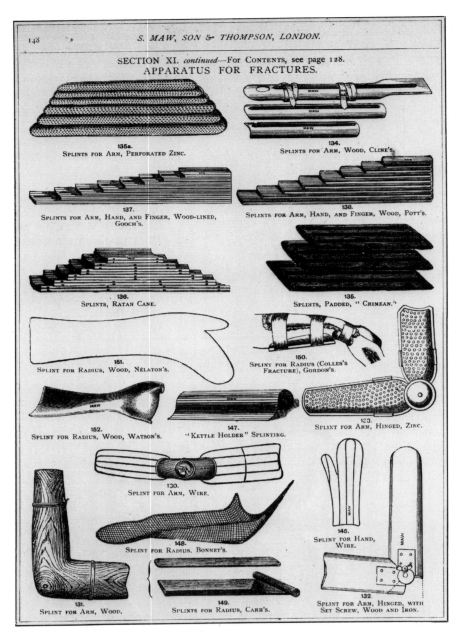

SECTION XI. *continued*—For CONTENTS, see page 128.
APPARATUS FOR FRACTURES.

135a.
SPLINTS FOR ARM, PERFORATED ZINC.

134.
SPLINTS FOR ARM, WOOD, CLINE'S.

137.
SPLINTS FOR ARM, HAND, AND FINGER, WOOD-LINED, GOOCH'S.

138.
SPLINTS FOR ARM, HAND, AND FINGER, WOOD, POTT'S.

136.
SPLINTS, RATAN CANE.

135.
SPLINTS, PADDED, " CRIMEAN."

151.
SPLINT FOR RADIUS, WOOD, NÉLATON'S.

150.
SPLINT FOR RADIUS (COLLES'S FRACTURE), GORDON'S.

152.
SPLINT FOR RADIUS, WOOD, WATSON'S.

147.
"KETTLE HOLDER" SPLINTING.

123.
SPLINT FOR ARM, HINGED, ZINC.

130.
SPLINT FOR ARM, WIRE.

145.
SPLINT FOR HAND, WIRE.

148.
SPLINT FOR RADIUS, BONNET'S.

131.
SPLINT FOR ARM, WOOD.

149.
SPLINTS FOR RADIUS, CARR'S.

132.
SPLINT FOR ARM, HINGED, WITH SET SCREW, WOOD AND IRON.

27. Apparatus for fracture management, *(from Maw's catalogue).*

On the other side was Hugh Owen Thomas who was educated in Edinburgh and University College Hospital, London. Thomas later practised at 11 Nelson Street, Liverpool, and was one of the founding members of the orthopaedic services in Liverpool. He had considerable ability in making splints, clinical skill and was a great exponent of rest which he suggested should be prolonged, uninterrupted and rigidly enforced.

Internal fixation of fractures was first attempted in Toulouse in 1770 and written up in the French *Journal of Surgery* in August 1775 by Lapuyode. A brass wire was used to hold a fractured humerus of a young boy. In 1912, further improvement in the technique of internal fixation was effected by Sir Arbuthnot Lane using a double plate for a humerus. However he had the problem of corrosion and infection.

Röntgen's discovery in the mid 1890's revolutionised the management of fractures by the use of X-rays. At the beginning of the twentieth century Albin Lambotte employed external fixation, using X-rays for the management of long bone fractures. He also appreciated the need for compression across a fracture site if he was going to use any form of internal fixation.

During the First World War, when large numbers of open fractures were sustained, the treatment was improved by the organisation of such casualties by Robert Jones who was a nephew of Hugh Owen Thomas. Further advances in the understanding of fracture union came with the work of Ernest Hey Groves. Born in 1872, he qualified initially as an engineer and later graduated in medicine from St Bartholomew's Hospital, London, in 1895. He practised originally in Bristol but commuted to University College Hospital in London to experiment on fracture union using cats and rabbits. He was fascinated by the operative treatment of fractures and showed that despite internal fixation non-union could happen. He wrote a treatise on the modern methods of treating fractures and suggested a use of bone pegs for non-union. He also suggested the use of transplantation of bone in the repair of defects. Bone transplants had been used by Ollier in 1867 and improved by Albee in 1915 but it was the work of Ernest Hey Groves which helped make grafting such a common feature today.

It is often said the rise of a speciality in medicine relates to the formation of an association and the publication of the scientific work of members of such an association. If so, orthopaedics became a separate entity on 28 November 1917 when a small number of surgeons met at the Café Royal in London. The result of this dinner was the formation of the British Orthopaedic Association. Ernest Hey Groves was one of the members present at that inaugural dinner. He became professor of surgery in Bristol in 1922, but it wasn't until the 1930's that Lord Nuffield inaugurated the first chair in orthopaedic surgery as a specific entity at Wingfield Morris Hospital, Oxford, and that chair was given to Gathorne Robert Girdlestone.

In the Spanish civil war Joseph Trueta gained great experience from the management of war casualties and suggested the use of plaster immobilisation of fractured femurs despite there being open injuries associated with such a fracture. He was to write extensively on the vascularity of bone and was later appointed to a chair in Oxford. Hoffman in the 1930's was an exponent of external fixation but it remained for Küntscher to suggest intra medullary nailing of long bones in 1942. Danis in Belgium in the 1940's used compression plates and he inspired Maurice Müller and Martin Allgöwer to formulate their principles of internal fixation. It is this Swiss school which today predominates in the Western world of internal fixation of fractures.

This short resumé shows that the management of fractures is both a craft and a science. Chaucer's quote from the *Comedy of Fools* remains as apt today as it did in the middle ages: "The life so short the craft so long to learn".

Acknowledgement

The author wishes to thank Mr C.L. Colton, FRCS for his help in the preparation of this paper.

Select Bibliography

1.   Walter G. Stuck, "Historic Background of Orthopaedic Surgery" *Ann Med. Hist.* 1935, **7**

2.   A.W. Beasley, "Orthopaedic Aspects of Medieval Medicine" *Jnl. Royal Society Medicine,* Dec.1982, **75**, pp 970-975

3.   A. W. Beasley, "Origins of Orthopaedics" *Jnl. Royal Society of Medicine,* Aug. 1982, **75**, pp 648-655.

4.   E. Bick, *Source Book of Orthopaedics*, Williams, Wilkins., 2nd.ed.1948.

Editorial note: In the *Medical Annual* of 1902 there is a reference to external fixation of two cases of un-united intracapsular fracture of the neck of the femur, usings pin of steel and ivory respectively. The reference given is 'Davis, *Univ. Med. Mag.*'

THE DENTAL PROFESSION IN THE PROVINCES IN THE 1850s

Christine Hillam

Professional toothdrawers seem to have been a normal part of European society from at least the middle ages. These men travelled around from market to market wearing distinctive hats and necklaces of teeth and adding their small mite to the sum total of human happiness.

Towards the end of the seventeenth century another group began to appear on the scene, the "operators for the teeth". As well as extracting, these men specialised in artificial replacements for lost teeth. Many appear to have emerged from the ranks of goldsmiths and metal workers.

In the early decades of the eighteenth century new elements were added to the treatment offered, namely restorative and preventive techniques. In fact by then work on the teeth embraced very much what is done today: treatment of the gums, fillings, crowns, bridges and artificial teeth, although the materials, of course, were different. Ivory, gold and lead were the order of the day, not polymers, amalgam and ceramics. A new name for the provider of these treatments also appeared. He now called himself a "dentist". This word originated in Italy as "dentista", became "chirurgien-dentiste" in France and surfaced as "dentist" in England in the 1750s.

This new group again emerged from the ranks of the goldsmiths and the jewellers and drew into its ambit such men as perfumers, barbers, patent medicine vendors and hairdressers. In England dentistry was not an offshoot or speciality of medicine. Nor was it aimed at the common man; the fees were too high. Twenty guineas was the usual charge for a full denture, a year's wages for an agricultural labourer. If ordinary people received any dental treatment at all, it was at the hands of the toothdrawer who co-existed with the dentist (albeit in sharply diminishing numbers) for a long time to come.

One may well ask why dentistry, this full range of preventive, restorative and prosthetic treatment, emerged precisely when it did. There is probably no one reason; the explanation lies more in the coincidence of a number of intertwining factors. Caries had been on the increase since the middle ages and had reached unprecedented levels by the mid-eighteenth century,[1] fuelled no doubt by the great increase in the consumption of sugar. Superimposed on this need was a change in social attitude towards rectifying the damage, closely related to the new idea of fashion which was part of the embryo consumer society. This was also the period when the new technology was looking for further outlets and when there was no shortage of entrepreneurial spirits ready to take up the challenge. Last but not least, there was a revolution in communications in the eighteenth century which was essential to the promotion of a new trade like dentistry. Since the market was so limited by economic considerations, early dentists, whether based in London or the provinces, regularly went on tours lasting a few weeks at a time in search of patients. To do this, they needed to make efficient use of the transport system and the advertising columns of the burgeoning provincial press, neither of which had reached a sufficient level of sophistication to make it worthwhile before the middle of the eighteenth century.

The Development of the Profession by the 1850s

In the century leading up to 1850, the idea of dentistry grew, although the numbers of resident dentists in the provinces remained very low indeed for the whole of the eighteenth and the beginning of the nineteenth centuries.[2] There were probably no more than twenty at any one time before 1810. After this date the number of dentists doubled approximately every ten years so that there were nearly 400 in 1850. A high rate of turnover meant that many more than this number were involved in the trade altogether. Of all the provincial practices set up before 1850, for example, about 30% survived no more than one year and about 40% no more than five years.

No. 10, Queen-Street, Queen-Square, Bath.
PRINCE, DENTIST.

ARTIFICIAL TEETH made on the moſt approved plan, which do not change their colour, have not any unpleaſant effect; and are ſo ſkilfully placed, from a ſingle one to a whole ſet, as not to be diſtinguiſhed from natural teeth.

Pure innocent Teeth placed to Stumps.

He has an eaſy method of concealing decayed Teeth in Front, ſo as not to be diſcovered they are decayed.

Teeth cleaned in the moſt pleaſing manner, and rendered white and beautiful, inſide as well as outſide.

Teeth drawn in the moſt careful manner.

Alſo fills up decayed Teeth, and performs all the various operations of the Teeth and Gums.

The real GERMAN CAKE of ROSES, which preſerves, faltens, and whitens the Teeth; deſtroys the Scurvy, and heals the Gums; makes the Lips of a healthy red, and ſweetens the Breath. It is ſo extremely pleaſant and innocent, that it might be uſed by infants.

Likewiſe, his LOTION, for cleaning Artificial Teeth, to be had as above.

28. Advertisement for Mr Prince, Dentist c1770.

A larger number of places were also involved by 1850. Resident dentistry had first appeared in the provinces in such places as the ports, the expanding cities with their merchant class and the watering places. By the period 1850-55 there were 165 places in provincial England and Wales sporting at least one resident dentist. The choice of location for a new practice was not related simply to the size of population. Although most new practices opened up in towns where there were already dentists, in every decade dentists set up business in places with surprisingly small populations, sometimes as low as 2,000, and the new manufacturing towns were generally ignored. Basically, the choice was related to wealth and a certain social attitude, which in the 1850s continued to reside more in the old centres than in the new. It also depended on personal preference; a Tavistock dentist explained in 1858 that he quite simply preferred to live in a small town rather than in a city, even though it meant him visiting a number of other similar towns regularly to earn a living.[3] City dentists also still went on their tours at this stage. It seems as though dentists belonged to an area rather than to a specific place and chose for the location of their practice the kind of place which suited their personal preferences, be it city or small country town.

Many of the very first dentists in the middle of the eighteenth century had originally been perfumers, hairdressers, barbers, patent medicine vendors, cuppers and bleeders, jewellers or watchmakers. A very few had been actors, already used to travelling the country in the practice of their profession. Another small group emanated from the medical profession (mostly from among the apothecaries). By 1850, these same groups were still entering dentistry at a mature age but the profession was drawing increasingly on school-leavers and on the sons of dental families.

At first, demand was low and some dentists (probably as many as 40%) undoubtedly continued to practice their old trade as well as their new one. The biggest group of part-time dentists were the chemists and druggists. From the beginning of the century this group had gradually been taking over the function of the professional toothdrawer and from the 1830s onwards a number began to offer the full range of treatments which constituted dentistry. However, by 1850, the vast majority of dentists were full-time and only about 15% of the new practices set up in the provinces in the early 1850s were worked part-time.

Despite a high turnover of dentists, those who persisted for more than ten years had careers every bit as long as their modern counterparts. They could also make a considerable amount of money. What evidence can be gleaned points to a gross of £700-£800 as being the norm[4] at a period when the majority of doctors in the provinces were earning only £200 or so.[5] They were also likely to leave estates worth two or even three times those of their contemporaries in medicine.[6] If we apply to them the criteria used by Brown in his study of medical men in Bristol in 1851,[7] then dentists can be seen as having a socio-economic status comparable with that enjoyed by the qualified surgeon or the Member of the Pharmaceutical Society.

Dentistry was a rapidly expanding activity in 1850 and yet there was no dental school in England until 1859, nor was there any institution for dentists comparable with the Royal Colleges or the Society of Apothecaries. There was no watertight legislation concerning education for dentistry until 1921 and certainly, in the 1850s, anyone was free to give dental practice a try as a means of earning a living. As James Robinson put it in 1844, "a brass plate and brazen impudence [were] all the diplomas necessary"[8] Many quite simply spent a few weeks or months learning the tricks of the trade from another dentist. Short training periods like this became a business sideline for some dentists. Some even operated a kind of franchise system, instructing a novice in the rudiments and then sending him out to practise in the firm's name, mechanical work to be sent back to base for processing.

Alongside these hasty graduates were those who served a three to five year apprenticeship to a practising dentist. The quality of their training depended on their master since there was no external body to regulate or monitor its content and there was little in the way of serious dental literature at the time to help the aspiring student. These trainees were likely to emerge from their apprenticeship well-versed in the mechanical side of dentistry but, according to some, without any systematic knowledge of the surgical aspect. They were, however, generally considered to make better dentists than those who studied surgery and then thought of dentistry as a career. The first such apprenticeships in the provinces date from the late eighteenth century. Because the majority post-date the apprenticeship tax records, it is impossible to say with certainty how many dentists trained by this method but the available evidence suggests that about half of those who made dentistry their career before the middle of the nineteenth century entered the profession by this route.

Finally, there were the dentists who set up practice after a number of years as an assistant or mechanic, learning on the job, having originally been an ivory turner or an instrument maker, perhaps. Conventional wisdom of the day accused them of being untrained and conversant only with the manufacture of dentures but there is ample evidence to show that many assistants were involved in clinical work. Unprincipled some of them certainly must have been, as in the case of Edward King, who broke away from his employer, Edward Lukyn of Oxford, to set up his own practice further down the High Street. Because King had signed a bond not to practice in the vicinity, he induced another dentist to come from London and set up the new business in *his* name. Gradually King absorbed most of the available custom and Lukyn had to move on to Leamington Spa.[9] But such rogues were probably the exception. On the surface of it, a dentist who started his own practice after 15-20 years as an assistant to another was probably better equipped for the dentistry of the day than a twenty year old just emerging from his formal apprenticeship.

With such a wide diversity of elements contained within the one blanket term "dentist", it is not perhaps surprising that self-interest predominated over unity. At the same time, the group had probably reached that stage in the life of any body where some organisation becomes inevitable, where boundaries have to be drawn, if only for the self-preservation of its most influential members.

The first hints at reform came in the late 1830s. In addition to the customary warnings in advertising booklets to beware of quacks, there appeared suggestions in the press that there should be a Faculty of Dentistry.[10] Perhaps with a sidelong look at the professionalising medical and pharmaceutical professions, in the 1840s attempts were made to interest both Parliament and the Royal College of Surgeons in dental reform,[11] to found a dental society[12] and to start dental journals.[13] This was to no avail, largely because of the inability of a few individuals to overcome the self-interest and inertia of the majority. The years around 1850 were the lull, or maybe the complacency, before the storm. For in 1855 a 22 year old dentist from Croydon called an open meeting of the profession which was to start off a far-reaching train of events.[14] From this sprang the College of Dentists, espoused to the cause of an independent profession. In reaction came the smaller Odontological Society (membership by invitation only), pinning its hopes on a more prestigious connection with the Royal College. Each inaugurated its own dental school and hospital to carry out its principles[15] and each had the editorial support of a new dental journal. A modification of its charter in September 1859 enabled the Royal College to grant a Licence in Dental Surgery, a triumph for the Odontological faction. The plan for an independent qualification was only finally abandoned by the College of Dentists in 1863 when the two rival groups buried the hatchet and amalgamated. The subsequent relationship between the dental and medical professions was an uneasy one, a problem not entirely resolved until the dental profession finally began to manage its own affairs in 1956.[16] One can only speculate how history would have taken a different course had the College of Dentists been triumphant in the middle of the last century.

The 1850s and the 1980s: Some Parallels

A comparison between the state of the dental profession in 1850 and in 1988 can be an instructive one, for in some respects events have turned full circle. After years of fighting for only registered dentists to work in the mouth, the profession now includes hygienists and therapists[17] and may also see one day denturists, former technicians who will be licensed to take impressions and make the resultant dentures. Gone are the days of the family concern (a feature of the second half of the last century); dentistry is once more seen as a safe profession in a volatile job market. As the respectable dentist of the past sought to distinguish himself from the ordinary practitioner by a licence, so there is now a proliferation of postgraduate qualifications, all of which undoubtedly further the interests of the patient and of science, but might also be seen as a self-protection mechanism operated by a profession feeling itself under pressure of numbers, as it did then. There has been a great surge in the last few years of private post-graduate courses, the publicity for which could almost have been written in the 1840s or 50s. Indeed, advertising is reappearing, to the same mixed reception that it aroused in the middle of the last century. When this is coupled with apparent increasing political pressure for dentistry to be excluded from the National Health Service, it seems very likely that the dentistry of the not-too-distant future may be characterised by competition between practitioners to provide some new, revolutionary treatment known only to them and care of the teeth will once more become a cosmetic extra instead of part of health care. In such an eventuality this would surely have an effect on the location of new practices; who would voluntarily go to an area of high unemployment when a professional income and job satisfaction were more likely to be attained where the wealth of the country was concentrated? *Plus ça change, plus c'est la même chose.*

29. Dental advertisements of the 1850s

MR. ALFRED HINTON,

Surgeon Dentist,

23, WALDON TERRACE,
TORQUAY.

Mr. H. supplies the loss of teeth, with all the most recent improvements, whereby the necessity of extracting the roots, or any other painful operation, is avoided.

Old sets re-fitted and rendered as serviceable as new.

Decayed Teeth made sound and preserved for many years by filling them with *gold sponge*, or a *soft white cement*, which in a few minutes becomes as hard as the tooth itself, and, in case the filling should at any future time fall out, Mr. H. will re-fill it without further charge.

Teeth extracted, with great care and safety, with instruments formed on the most modern and scientific principles, preventing much needless pain.   Children's Teeth regulated during their second dentition, so as to insure a future healthy and regular set.

A single mineral Tooth, of the best quality, colour, and shape, and which will never wear out, from 8s.

Teeth cleaned and scaled, or made firm in their sockets, 3s. 6d. Decayed Teeth filled, 2s. 6d. If more than one, at a reduced charge.

Teeth filled for servants, 1s. 6d.   Extracted, 1s.   Nerve destroyed without pain, 1s. 6d.

Mr. H. conducts his practice on honourable principles, and will return the amount paid by any patient, who, after a fair trial, shall feel dissatisfied.

. . . and the 1980s.

Clinical Foundation
of
Orthopaedics & Orthodontics

INTERCEPTIVE ORTHODONTICS
and FUNCTIONAL THERAPY

Worried by delays in obtaining help for your patient's orthodontic problems?

**On SATURDAY/SUNDAY, MARCH 21/22, at the
GATWICK PENTA Hotel.**

Dr J. W. TRUITT, BS.DDS. will be presenting a two day seminar which will allow you to diagnose and treat most of the malocclusions which you see in your practice, even though you have little previous experience.

Course Fee £225. which includes lunches and refreshments on seminar days, and all materials needed.

Further Information/Bookings:-
**Mr. P. Hett, 68 St. Peters Avenue,
Cleethorpes, Lincolnshire DN35 8HP
Tel. 0472 691708**

(15

REFERENCES AND NOTES

1.   See a series of papers by W.J. Moore and M.E. Corbett, "The distribution of dental caries in ancient British populations", *Caries Research*, **5**, 1971, pp 151-168; **7**, 1973, pp 139-153; **9**, 1975, pp 163-175; **10**, 1976, pp 401-414

2.   Statements made about numbers of dentists, places, turnover etc, are based on F.C. Hillam, "The development of dental practice in the provinces from the late 18th century to 1855" (unpublished PhD thesis, University of Liverpool, 1986)

3.   "Suaviter et fortiter, Quackery and country practice", *British Journal of Dental Science*, **2**, 1858, p 49

4.   e.g. advertisement for the sale of a practice (*Brit.J.dent. Sci*, **1**, 1856-57, p 197) and cash books of James Prew of Bath, Wellcome Library, MS 5208-5214

5.   J.C. Hudson, *The parents' handbook - or guide to the choice of employments, professions, etc*, London, 1842

6.   Based on a survey of probate records of 262 provincial dentists in practice for more than ten years before 1855

7.   P.S. Brown, "The providers of medical treatment in mid-nineteenth century Bristol", *Med. Hist*, **24**, 1980, pp 297-314

8.   *Forceps*, **1**, 1844-45, p 62

9.   *ibid*, p 98

10.   e.g. *Lancet*, 1840-41, p 898

11.   G. Waite, *An appeal to Parliament, the medical profession and the public, on the present state of dental surgery*, London, 1841

12.   T. Purland, *Dental memoranda* 1844, p 122v: a letter from James Robinson inviting him to form the British Society of Dental Surgeons (Wellcome Library, MS 63518)

13.   James Robinson had been editor of two short-lived dental periodicals, *British Quarterly Journal of Dental Science*, 30 Mar-30 June 1843 and *Forceps*, (13 Jan 1844-Dec 1845)

14.   Samuel Lee Rymer (1833-1909)

15.   The Odontological Society founded the Dental Hospital of London (Nov 1858) and the London School of Dental Surgery (1859); the College of Dentists had its Metropolitan School of Dental Science (June 1859) and the National Dental Hospital (Nov 1861)

16.   The General Dental Council was established in 1956

17.   Trained for a maximum of two years

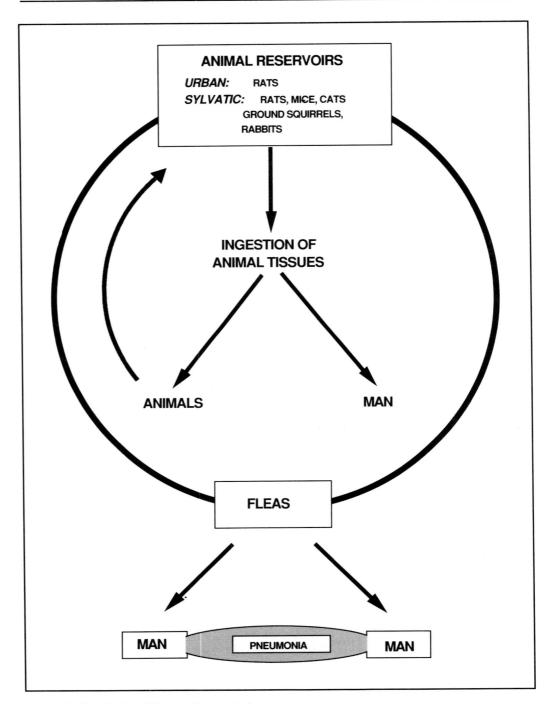

Figure 3. The Cycle of Plague Transmission

SEARCHING FOR PLAGUE IN SOMERSET

Nigel Lightfoot and James Skeggs

This work arose out of a meeting of a consultant medical microbiologist and the Accessions Officer of Somerset Record Office. Using our respective skills of an understanding of the disease plague and an understanding of the use of records we have pursued the history of plague in the rural county of Somerset. The factors affecting the transmission of plague are discussed and examples of recorded plague events between 1538 and 1666 are presented. Plague certainly occurred in Somerset but its impact does not appear to have been great.

It must be remembered that plague is primarily and was primarily a disease of rats. It is a zoonotic infection caused by the bacterium *Yersinia pestis* and is transmitted among the natural animal reservoirs through vector flea bites or occasionally by the ingestion of contaminated animal tissues. The animal reservoirs may be urban or sylvatic rodents (i.e. living in cities or in the country).

Although the term *plague* refers specifically to the disease caused by the organism *Yersinia pestis*, in common usage it often means any infectious disease and implies the capacity of that disease to spread through the human population at a rapid rate.

We are currently experiencing the fourth great pandemic in the world. The previous three are believed to have occurred in the following times.[1] The first originated in Egypt in 542 A.D. and spread to Turkey and Europe. The second pandemic started in the fourteenth century in Asia Minor and Africa and after spreading to Europe killed about a quarter of that continent's population. The third also occurred in Europe during the fifteenth to eighteenth centuries.

The present pandemic that we are experiencing began in Yunnan in China in 1860, spread to the southern coast of China reaching Hong Kong in 1894, where Yersin and Kitasato discovered the causative organism. Subsequently, plague was carried by ships and their rats to India, other countries of Asia, to Brazil, and even to California.

Transmission of Plague

Throughout the world the urban and domestic rats *Rattus rattus* and *Rattus norvegicus* are the most important reservoirs of the plague bacillus. Man is an accidental host in the natural cycle of infection when he is bitten by a rodent flea. Man appears to play no part in the maintenance of *Yersinia pestis* in nature, and only rarely during epidemics of pneumonic plague is the infection believed to be passed directly from man to man. Rarely man may also develop infection by the direct handling of contaminated animal tissues, although this is now the main route of transmission in California and the Middle East.

The occurrence of human plague is nearly always linked to the transmission of plague among the natural animal reservoirs. The incidence of plague in humans is therefore a function of both the frequency of infection, local rodent population and the intimacy with which people live with the infected rodents and their fleas.

In the entire history of urban human plague the domestic black rat *Rattus rattus* has probably been the most important host. This rat lives in close association with man and inhabits ships as well as houses. It is the host for the efficient plague flea vector *Xenopsylla cheopis*. Plague in rural settings, however, has taken on many complex variations. The classic theory of plague reservoirs requires one or more relatively resistant small mammal species which serve as the enzootic reservoir and one or more relatively susceptible species which serve as the epizootic host and may be involved in the so-called rat die-offs or rat falls. The rat generally lives for just under one year and may not always be killed by the infection. The brown rat has almost completely replaced the black rat in modern times such that the black rat now only occurs around port areas. There are even recent reports suggesting that it may have disappeared altogether. The brown rat does not live in as close association with man; it lives in farm buildings and hedgerows away from human habitation. Its flea, *Nosopsylla ceratophyllus fasciatus* really does not like biting man and this may explain in part why plague disappeared from the Western world.

The commission for the investigation of plague in India established that the oriental rat flea *Xenopsylla cheopis* was the most important vector of plague transmission. The reason why this was an efficient vector was shown by Bacot and Martin in 1914.[2] They demonstrated that several days after ingesting infective rat blood the proventriculus of these fleas became obstructed by a solid mass of plague bacteria. These fleas became "blocked" so that subsequent blood feedings could not pass into the stomach. Nevertheless, the blocked fleas tried to feed and regurgitated blood, which was contaminated by their own bacteria in the obstructed proventriculus, back into the wound. Not satisfying their thirst, they made repeated bites. Through this blocking mechanism *Xenopsylla cheopis* was a more efficient vector than other rat fleas. The blocked fleas eventually died, their survival time being influenced by temperature and humidity but being about 21 days.

The blocking of fleas by *Yersinia pestis* appears to be very important in the transmission of plague but transmission by other methods might have occurred. For instance, the penetration of infected flea faeces into abraded skin and the mechanical transmission through biting with infected flea mouth parts may play a part.

Although the common route of human transmission is from infected rodent fleas, outbreaks of plague pneumonia spread by infected air-borne droplets or aerosols have occurred. Fortunately, this mode of man-to-man transmission is rare and seems to be very short lived; because plague pneumonia is so rapidly fatal victims have little time to spread their infection to others. They rapidly became prostrate and die within 24 hours.

The potential of a human reservoir was suggested by Marshall and co-workers in Vietnam who demonstrated the oral carrier state.[4] The pharyngeal carrier state persisted for as long as 21 days. None of these carriers developed pneumonic plague and there was no evidence that they were contagious. However, these studies point out the alarming possibility of a silent human reservoir from which pneumonic plague epidemics could erupt.

Another form of inter-human transmission, directly by fleas, has been observed in Kurdish peoples by Blanc and Blatazard. They presented evidence that the human flea, *Pulex irritans*, may transmit the disease from man to man.[5] This mode of transmission is rare and requires extremely unhygienic and crowded living conditions. This could have obviously occurred in ancient epidemics. In fact, this sort of historical presentation has been advanced by Ell for the mediaeval plague epidemics.[6] According to this argument, human flea transmission rather than either rat flea or respiratory droplet transmission should be associated with the interpersonal spread of human plague and should result in large number of cases per household in the absence of rat mortality.

Clinical Features

Following the bite of an infected flea the bacteria proliferate in the lymph nodes that drain the area and, after two to eight days, there is a sudden onset of fever, chills, weakness and headache. The patient will feel quite ill and some four to twenty-four hours later a lymphatic swelling occurs. This is known as a bubo and may be accompanied by redness and swelling. Septicaemia can occur some twenty-four hours later with a spill-over of the organisms from the lymph nodes into the blood stream. There will then be severe prostration with restlessness. A purpuric rash has been noticed on occasions which may lead to necrosis or gangrene. Often the septicaemia, if untreated, will result in death but, if the recovery occurs, the patient will be immune. Later pus will often drain from the bubo.

The clinical features of plague are typical but it should be remembered that buboes can be caused by several other diseases that were present at that time. Included in the differential diagnosis are secondary syphilis, lymphogranuloma venereum, granuloma inguinale and abscesses due to *Staphylococcus aureus* and *Streptococcus pyogenes*.

In a few cases following the septicaemia a plague pneumonia may develop and, at this stage, the organisms proliferate in the lungs and may be coughed up into an exhaled aerosol which may be infective to others. This can produce secondary inhalation pneumonic plague. In modern outbreaks this has been found to be rare and because death usually ensues within twenty-four hours and the patient is often prostrate it is suggested that a patient with pneumonic plague would have very little time to spread it to his fellow man.

The Occurrence of a Plague Outbreak

The infection must first of all be established in rats having been brought to them by other rats or by sylvatic rodents. The epidemic in rats will cause them to die and their fleas will leave the rat carcass and look for an alternative source of food. If the rats are in close association with man the fleas will then feed on him. Man will then almost certainly become infected with plague but, as we have suggested before, man-to-man transmission is extremely rare. If we are to search for plague among historical records we must consider those things that may point to a plague outbreak; a rat die-off will certainly indicate plague occurring amongst those animals and because the disease is so typical clinical descriptions of cases may be extremely helpful. We can also look for records specifically mentioning plague; we have therefore searched in the parish records and Quarter Sessions rolls for evidence of plague infection in Somerset.

During this period there was common and almost unrelieved pain from infected wounds, bad teeth and gastric troubles associated with infected or badly prepared, or decaying food. By comparison with todays conditions, life was hard and comfortless, a great part of the population was surviving at subsistence level, and there was a high birth and death rate. The limited diet was deficient in vitamins A and D, perhaps causing stones in the bladder and urinary tract as well as blindness. Periods of famine and prolonged bad weather produced outbreaks of scurvy and made conditions ideal for other diseases including plague.[7]

In earlier times, plague had an aura of mystery - the wrath of God being one of the usually attributed causes. The methods of control were often quarantine - reaching a peak with the Act 1 Jac. cap. 31 making it a felony to go abroad and converse in company whilst infected by the plague[8] - and remedies approaching witchcraft. During this period there were many forms of amulet used against disease.

Examinations of the Bills of Mortality (from c 1532) which show the causes of death in the City of London, produce such cases as ague, fever, flux and smallpox as well as plague. These diagnoses were achieved by "ancient matrons sworn to their office" who "repair to the place where the dead corpse lies and by view of the same ... examine by what disease ... the corpse died".[9] Some doubt can therefore be put upon those statistics! Here it may be amusing to consider one Dr Thompson who applied to his stomach a large dried toad sewn up in a linen cloth "where after it had remained for some hours .. became ... so distended ... that it was an object of wonder to those who believed it".[10]

The hypotheses of well-known writers who give the impression that the plague swept the country like wild-fire, killing half the population and leaving masses of evidence in records and folk memory, have to be reconsidered in a balanced way, for in our part of the country, such written evidence is thin on the ground, and folk memory proves, in reality, mainly to be eighteenth and nineteenth century romanticism. Plague years: Although there is clearly some evidence that there were epidemics in some years, not all cases described as plague relate to Bubonic Plague. Specific records of plague deaths are limited to say the least, and not all cases so described can be definitely diagnosed as such. Except for the known cases of plague in the larger towns and the Eyam outbreak, we have no definite information of rural occurrence of Bubonic Plague, and have to ask ourselves if we are dealing with other infectious diseases. There is however one such occurrence in Somerset:

Memorandum. That in Anno Domini 1645 in the parish of East Coker from the 8 day of June until the 10 day of September there died and were interred in the contagious sickness, plague and pestilence, threescore and ten persons - and so it pleased the Almighty, suddenly beyond all men's expectation, to put an end to this fearful visitation - for which extraordinary favour we ascribe all laud and praise unto His Sacred Name.

So reads a sad entry in East Coker's burial register.[11]

Records of Plague Events

In enquiring into any event using archival material, it is essential to establish sources and parameters within which to work. We decided to use three main sources, and to discuss the years between 1538 and 1666. Those sources are:

Parish Registers

Thomas Cromwell, Lord Chancellor, ordered in 1538 a register to be kept in each parish church of all baptisms, marriages and burials. This ensured a proper registration system which, with minor exceptions, remained unchanged until the nineteenth century. Thus those registers which survived the ensuing 450 years of war, famine, fire, vermin and careless vicars have ensured a vast reservoir of statistical information. With hindsight, Cromwell should have included ages and causes of death to help us along the road in our small study! Here we must add that our inquiry has so interested us, we have embarked on a systematic study of death statistics in this county, parish by parish.

The few definite mentions of plague in registers are quite clear. In the village of West Buckland, there is a record of burials in fields.[12] At Taunton St Mary[13] the left hand margin of the register is marked clearly to indicate plague burials, and the same can be seen at High Ham,[14] whilst at Minehead[15] there are group burials which may indicate contagious disease deaths. In other cases, the times when plague struck and ended have been noted, for example at Pilton,[16] and at Lower Weare.[17]

Records of Quarter Sessions

These are the court records which have handed down to us a wealth of information on Local Government affairs, and in the case of our particular study, the levying of rates to pay the expenses of putting into quarantine a family from London who came to visit friends at Frome in 1625.[18]

Another example shows that in Yeovil[19] four men had been persuaded to carry out the burial of the dead at a time when the contagion was so serious that many died, and no-one would act as gravedigger. They did the work, but payment was not forthcoming, and so they petitioned the court for their money two years after the event, *i.e.* in 1647. A final example, from Minehead,[20] is the petition of a man who had disbursed monies for the victualling and relief of poor persons infected with the plague, but could not get reimbursement without going to court for it. This was in 1619.

Among other cases, we have found one really good example from the tiny parish of Compton Pauncefoot[21] (illustration 30), which details the full story of an infectious disease in one family. The main point at issue appears to be that the householder not only invited people into his home, but went out into the countryside. We have a description of the malady as well. His daughter was infected, died, and upon view "it was found that her bodie was spotted over a great part". This may however indicate smallpox or

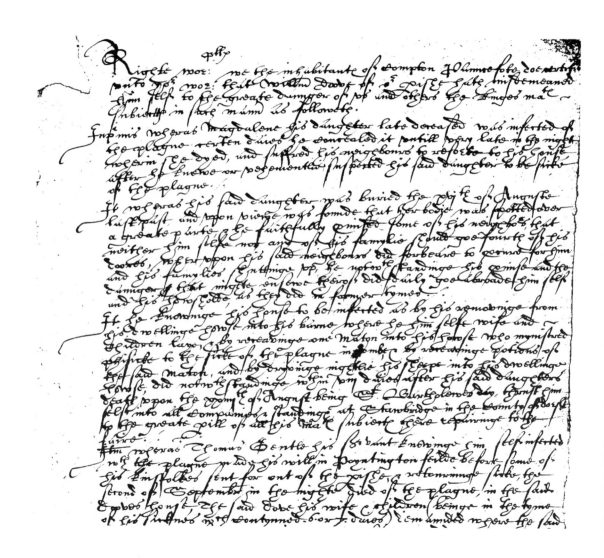

30. Quarter Sessions Rolls of 1611 describing plague in Compton Pauncefoot.

the "Spotted fever" - *i.e.* typhus. His servant died a few days later, but the parish register[22] simply records the burials and makes no mention of disease. This is another example of how little can be deduced from basic statistics. Both had different names, and there is no mention of an infection, so the register gives us no idea that the cases were either related or had any connection with plague. There is, however, an indication in the Rolls of an attempt at remedial precautions. The man moved his family from the house into his barn, and drove his sheep into the house every night. To any one who has had dealings with sheep, this can only mean that he knew the pungency of sheep's urine, and the Somerset belief that it is a disinfectant which will kill or disturb vermin.

Meteorological Records

These help provide us with an understanding of tolerable conditions, year by year, for famine, plague and therefore the times of unfavourable conditions for humans. They consequently lead us to appreciate the years favourable to the Black Rat.

Geographical Considerations

Somerset's maritime position

Somerset has a long coastline which contains ports. Ports have ships in them. Ships carry rats perhaps more efficiently than any other vehicle. We can consider the following places as important points of embarkation of infected rodents: Bristol, Avonmouth, Bridgwater, Watchet, Minehead and Porlock.[23]

The Somerset plain and levels

Three hundred years ago this was an area of marsh, swamp and generally difficult terrain, hindering the movement of people, but more especially our little rodents. On the other hand, it provided super opportunities for diseases like the ague and malaria to breed with impunity. Here we would do well to read Peter Franklin's paper on malaria in mediaeval Gloucestershire.[24]

The inherent quality of life in rural Somerset

There was a balanced and fair distribution of vermin as matter of course, and the well-known laws in sixteenth and seventeenth century England relating to the destruction and/or capture thereof which have extended into modern times, especially regarding rats. Nowadays the rodent officer is called out to deal with the occasional wasps' or hornets' nest, but by far the greatest call on his time, even today, is the destruction of the rat. This is one great example of folk fear of the wicked ghost of the Pied Piper, though time has transposed the Black Rat into Brown.

Towns were small, and the houses therein even smaller than we care to contemplate. Consider Taunton, where the town gates were by modern standards close to each other, and the now fashionable church of Wilton was once in a village way beyond the town boundaries. In village communities, the population was scattered, and the housing, and consequently the sanitary conditions were of poor quality. Vermin destruction took place with an exactitude which we find difficult to believe today - for in that destruction lay the success of good husbandry.

31. Excerpt from the Bradford on Tone Parish Register. 1525.

Civil war and famine

Following hard upon the upheaval of the dissolution of the monasteries and the subsequent administrative chaos came the period of great wealth of the later part of the Elizabethan age, when the lot of the average man must have improved considerably, especially in regard to health and hygiene. In fact life generally became so good, as compared with that enjoyed by previous generations, that the inevitable reaction was to come from the grass-roots of our English politics in its infancy - the wish to condemn the autocracy of our fore-fathers, the old ways and the slackness in religious zeal. The King (Charles I) disagreed with his countrymen, and so followed civil war on a scale previously unknown to the English. Hard on the tracks of the soldiers came the famine, pestilence and hunger known to follow armies since recorded history began.

Conclusions

Did we find Bubonic Plague in Somerset? It is fair to conclude that in the larger towns we did, but that other illnessses were also very much in evidence. Again we cite the case of typhus or smallpox in Compton Pauncefoot. It should also be noted that there was an outbreak of dysentery in Minehead in 1596, shown in the parish registers as The Bloody Flux.[25] Were it not for this note by the parish priest, we could be forgiven for thinking that this was plague. There can therefore be seen the danger of jumping to conclusions.

Finally, there is an entry in the village register for Bradford on Tone,[26] when the vicar of this small village buried his wife (illustration 31). Freely translated it says that she died of the pestilence, then adds "may it not touch me!". There were many contagious and virulent diseases at large, not understood in the sixteenth and seventeenth centuries, which as far as the population at that time was concerned, were unable to be accounted for, took away their loved ones, and were in every sense a plague.

ACKNOWLEDGEMENTS

We should particularly like to thank Derek Shorrocks, lately Somerset County Archivist, and his successor, Adam Green, for their kind help and permission to reproduce material in the Somerset Record Office. Our thanks are also due to Gwen Chapman who typed the manuscript several times and helped considerably with the layout.

REFERENCES

Abbreviations used in subsequent freferences:

Somerset Record Office (SRO) deposited documents:

D/P/   Parish collections
Q/S   Quarter sessions records
Q/SR   Quarter sessions rolls (Roll number, folio and date)

1.   L G Lipson, "Plague in San Francisco in 1900: The United States Marine Hospital Service Commission to study the existence of plague in San Francisco". *Ann Intern Med* 1972. **77**:pp 303-310

2.   A W Bacot, C J Martin, "Observations on the mechanism of the transmission of plague by fleas". *J Hyg* 1914. **13**:pp 432-439

3.   J H Rust, D C Cavanaugh, R O'Shita and J D Marshall, "The role of domestic animals in the epidemiology of plague. 1. Experimental Infection of dogs and cats." *J Infect Dis* 1971. **124**:pp 522-526

4.   J D Marshall, D V Quy and F L Gibson, "Asymptomatic pharyngeal plague infection in Vietnam". *Am J Trop Med Hyg* 1967. **16**:pp 175-177

5.   G Blanc and M Baltazhard, "Recherches sur la mode de transmission naturelle de la peste bubonique et septicemique". *Arch Inst Pasteur Maroc* 1945. **3**:pp 175-354

6.   S R Ell, "Some evidence for interhuman transmission of mediaeval plague". *Rev Infect Dis* 1979 **1**(3):pp 563-566

7.   J M Stratton and J H Brown, *Agricultural Records, A.D. 220-1977*, John Baker, 1969

8.   W Lee and D Pakeman, *Institute of the Laws of England*, J Flesher, London, 1660

9.   J Graunt, *Natural and Political Observations ... made upon the bills of mortality*, London, 1662

10.   G Thompson, *Loimotomia, or the pest anatomised*, London, 1666; Philip Ziegler, *The Black Death*, Collins, 1969

11.   SRO   D/P/cok.e. 2/1/1

12.   SRO   D/P/w.bu. 2/1/1

13.   SRO   D/P/tau.m 2/1/1

14.   SRO   D/P/ham.h. 2/1/1

15.   SRO   D/P/m.st.m. 2/1/1

16.   SRO   D/P/pilt 2/1/1

17.   SRO   D/P/wea. 2/1/1

18.   SRO   Q/SR 56/ii/51 - 1625

19.   SRO   Q/SR 80/21 - 1647

20.   SRO   Q/SR 32/i/32 - 1619

21.   SRO   Q/SR 14/88 - 1611

22.   SRO   D/P/comp.p. 2/1/1

23.   Stratton and Brown, op. cit.

24.   Peter Franklin, Malaria in Mediaeval Gloucestershire - an essay in epidemiology, *Transactions of the Bristol and Gloucestershire Archaeological Society,* **101,** 1983

25.   SRO   D/P/m.st.m. 2/1/1

26.   SRO   D/P/bra.t. 2/1/1

COLICA PICTONUM: Taking the Cure in Bath

Audrey Heywood

A concise description of the Colica Pictonum was given by Dr Rice Charleton[1] one of the senior Physicians at the Bath Hospital in his *Tract on the Bath Waters* published in 1770.

"In consequence of a most obstinate costiveness attended with exquisite pain in the bowels, upon the constipation being removed and the pain diminished, the patient loses the use of his limbs. The arms and hands most commonly. Rheumatic pains sometimes attack the limbs before they become paralytic."

The colic which gives rise to this species of palsy was not unknown to the ancients. It was twice mentioned by Paulus Aegina in the seventh century.

This was the syndrome or pattern of symptoms described by Citius[2], Cardinal Richelieu's physician, in 1616 when he called it the *Colica Pictonum*. Although there had been widespread epidemics of colic followed by palsy for centuries there was no clear idea of the cause of this disorder. It was attributed to anything from metallic poisons or unresolved fevers to over-indulgence in acid wines, high living or passions of the mind. Sir George Baker's classic work on *The Devonshire Colic*[3] published in 1767 established that lead was the cause of the *Colica Pictonum* and that the Devonshire colic, *Huttenkatze* and the West Indian Dry Gripes were the same disease.

Lead poisoning had been a widespread but undiagnosed problem from Roman times until the end of the nineteenth century. A large proportion of the population would have been affected to some degree. Any population using lead pipes to carry soft water, lead glazed earthenware containers for food and drink, cooking pots tinned with the usual mixture of tin and lead, pewter plates and tankards and lead lined sinks and storage boxes could readily acquire a significant lead load. Cosmetics were often lead based as were food colorants, and lead salts were frequently used medicinally.

For many people this level of poisoning would have caused tiredness, headaches and a vague feeling of malaise, but others were more seriously affected. These were the people who added to their base load of lead repeated doses of comparatively small amounts of lead from occupational exposure or lead adulterated alcohol.

This retrospective study has been possible because this more serious severe lead poisoning presented in such a readily recognisable and characteristic way. The connection between Bath spa therapy and the *Colica Pictonum* had started long before the founding of the Hospital in the eighteenth century.

As early as the beginning of the sixteenth century Bath had a well established reputation for curing people with paralyses — its collection of discarded crutches had become legendary.[4] But some cases did better than others, particularly those patients with paralyses that followed attacks of severe griping abdominal pain. They called this "The

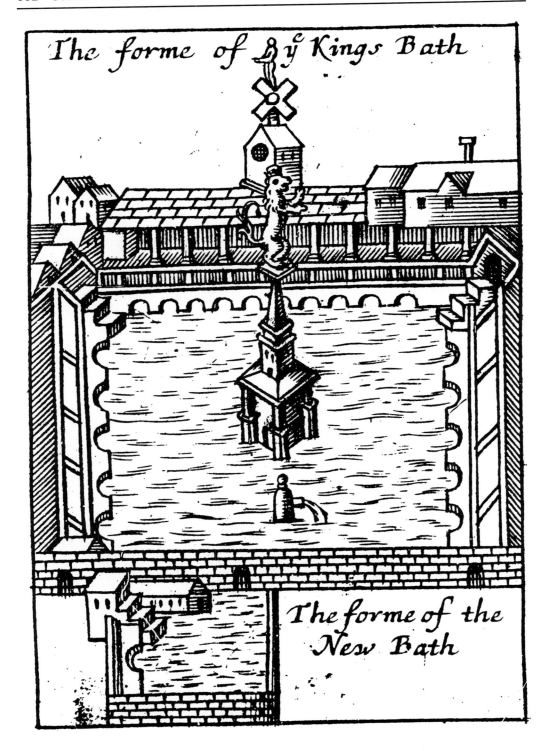

The forme of ꝑ y Kings Bath

The forme of the
New Bath

palsy after the Colic". In 1713 Dr. Robert Pierce[5] published his memoirs of sixty years of practice as the senior physician in Bath. He recorded and classified most of the cases he had seen from the middle of the seventeenth century onward.

Because he was so familiar with many types of paralysis he was able to differentiate "the Palsy after the Colic" from the paralyses that were "the consequence of Apoplexes, Epilepsies or Convulsions" and identified it as the *Colica Pictonum*. He found "no one Distemper more frequent amongst my Adversaria, nor in none more eminent recoveries than in this or persons thus disabled, to have been restored by the assistance of the Bath and the Bath waters". His patients came from as far afield as the West Indies, Ireland, the Channel Isles and East Anglia.

The generally accepted, conventional treatment which was used in Europe and the Americas[6] consisted of emetics and purges. Opiates were added if the pain was very severe. Taken early enough this was often sufficient to cure the colic but if a paralysis subsequently developed, continued purging together with a bland diet, weak beer to drink and removal from the work environment usually cured that as well. Sometimes, however, the paralysis persisted or became more widespread; this was a disaster as the man could no longer earn his living.[7] It was to these patients, who had often been disabled for many months, that the cures obtained in Bath must have seemed so remarkable. In addition to the usual treatments there was the use of the copious supply of hot mineral waters. The Bath waters were widely acknowledged to be the most effective treatment for all these persistent cases.

A pattern for bathing and drinking the water had gradually evolved. People usually bathed in the morning; since Tudor times the water had been changed daily so the baths were closed from noon to allow this to take place. The earliest bathers had the cleanest water. Even so Samuel Pepys[8] was astonished to find fashionable people bathing in the Cross Bath at 5 am.

Celia Fiennes[9] noted on her visit in 1687 that the bathers stood or sat up to the neck in water. Stone "coushons" were provided for those who found the seats too low. Bathing could last from a half to several hours and music and other entertainments were provided to pass the time.

Drinking the water became more acceptable after 1650 when a clean supply direct from the source was provided. About 1-2 pints were consumed each morning in divided doses, sometimes more. By 1700 it was common knowledge that Bath was the place to go to if you were left with a palsy after an attack of severe colic. So the Bath physicians saw many cases and recognised this highly characteristic disease, knowing that they could cure many of these patients. But other doctors were doubtful of these claims. By then more than anecdotal evidence was needed to prove the curative powers of "the Bath Waters". It was felt that by setting up a charity hospital, the doctors could provide good support for their claims in a very modern and scientific way.

32. (left) The Kings Bath in the early 17th century. *(J. Speed).*

Regulating the treatment and allowing adequate time to achieve the best possible results provided valuable evidence of the efficacy of the Bath spa treatment. As the final outcome of treatment would be assessed by a committee of doctors, not only the one in charge of the case, no charge of bias could be brought.

Thus by recording the results it would be possible to provide "irrefutable proof" of the curative powers of the Bath waters. The idea of founding a charity hospital was first considered in 1723 but it was not possible to raise the necessary funds. When it was successfully relaunched in 1737 the *Design for the Bath Hospital*[10] stated:

"All physicians allow that the greatest certainty that can be attained to in the knowledge of the Natures and Virtue of any Medicine arises out of the number of observations of the effect it has on Human Bodies in Different Circumstances ......but surely if the Knowledge of the Nature and Efficacy of these Waters could still be rendered more extensive and certain it would be doing a great service to every individual Person."

The Bath Hospital opened its doors in 1741. The patients were carefully selected; only those who would benefit from the special treatment in Bath were admitted. A referral letter had to be sent and these letters were vetted by a group of Doctors to make sure that the patients were "suitable Objects for Charity". The poor accepting treatment agreed to stay until the physicians considered that they were cured or improved as much as possible. In return the hospital provided accommodation, a good diet and additional medications if needed and the use of the mineral waters, i.e. spa therapy *sans* glamour for the deserving poor. On discharge these charity patients were seen by the committee of doctors who decided on the final diagnosis and outcome of treatment. It was clearly stated that no one was to be considered to be cured if any sign of the original disorder remained.

All this information was recorded together with length of stay and personal details, at first in the Minute Book[11], together with a copy of the referral letter. The physicians were required to keep good records and to publish their findings. Because it was a charity hospital an Annual Report[11] was published each year.

On being admitted the patients were removed from their normal environment and from the source of lead pollution. They were provided with adequate fresh food which was cheap and plentiful in Bath. There was also a supply of home-brewed beer. Drinking outside the hospital was banned. Patients were given preparatory medication if required, usually purges.

Bathing was carried out three days a week, (Dr. Summers said for over an hour), usually in the Hot Bath which had been allocated to the charity patients. However, on the occasions when the cooler Cross Bath was used both Dr. Summers in 1751 and Dr. Falconer[12] in the 1790's remarked that they achieved cures more rapidly. In 1830 when the hospital got its own bath the temperature was kept at about 35°C. The patients drank about 1-1 pints of water a day in divided doses. Pumping water onto the paralysed limb was also thought to be helpful in the convalescent stages.

A sophisticated, scientific trial of the Bath Waters had been designed and we have evidence from the records kept in the hospital that the protocol laid down was carefully observed.

A picture painted in 1741 of Dr. Oliver and Mr. Pierce, the surgeon, examining patients together still hangs in the main hall of the hospital. This demonstration of the diagnostic committee in action was important as the committee played an essential part in establishing the reliability of the trial. Dr Summers wrote[13] "when patients are discharged it is what the whole committee sees and examines which is recorded. It is therefore a Testimony to be relied on."

The findings of the committee were recorded in the Minute Book. The entry for April 6th 1754 shows that a Sam Ariss was admitted on 8th November 1753. He had been examined by Dr. Abel Moysey (A.M.) and Mr. F. Palmer (F.P.) who had decided that he had had *Colica Pictonum* but was cured. This information about individual patients was also recorded together with a copy of the referral letter in the Referral Register. From that entry we know that Sam Ariss was a 25 year old journeyman painter from Birmingham, who had had a weakness in his hands since Christmas 1752 and had been unable to work since then.

The results of the analysis of the only surviving Referral Register from May 1751 - 1758 show that of the 1590 cases admitted during that period 108 had symptoms of chronic lead poisoning. These 108 cases fell into two distinct groups, 37 in which there was evidence of occupational exposure, and 71 in which there was a clear history of a peripheral paralysis following an attack or several attacks of severe colic but no definite history of lead exposure.

The group with occupational exposure (31 patients, 6 readmissions) contained 11 painters, 7 plumbers, 4 glaziers, 5 lead manufacturers, 2 glass grinders, 1 potter and 1 gilder. On discharge, 22 (59%) were cured and a total of 34 (93%) were improved after an average stay of 149 days. Twenty came from London or the south east. Fifteen of these patients had been referred from London hospitals as incurable but after treatment in Bath, eight were cured and the other seven improved. These results support the view that the treatment in Bath had something special to offer, as in London they would have been removed from exposure to lead, given purges, emetics and a bland diet to no avail.

The other group with no definite exposure to lead presented with the classical symptoms of the Devonshire colic:- colic followed by paralysis.

More patients, 43 of 71, came from the south west than in the previous group and had a longer stay in the hospital, 168 days on average. Compared to the cases due to occupational exposure, a smaller proportion (42%) of cases were cured although a total of 93% were improved.

In 1760 Dr. Rice Charleton was able to classify the results. Outcome fell into six groups:- Cured, Much Improved, No Better, Improper (unsuitable for treatment) Irregular, (discharged before the treatment was completed for misbehavour or at their own request) or Dead. The patients were also put into seven diagnostic categories: Rheumatism, Paralysis, Leprosy or skin disease, Lameness, Hip cases and Jaundice. A year later Paralysis due to *Colica Pictonum* was added.

In 1770 Dr Rice Charleton, in *Three tracts on the Bath waters*, listed cases seen by himself and Dr. William Oliver. His publication included the table; "A State of the paralytic Patients admitted into the Bath Hospital, from May 1751, to May 1764." The total number of cases admitted was 1053 of which 813 were cured or benefited by the treatment in the hospital. Of 237 cases admitted with "Palsies from Cyder and Bilious Cholics", 218 were said to have benefited. (92%). Of the 40 patients with palsies due to metallic effluvia, 38 benefited. (95%).

Clearly the hospital physicians considered that the treatment of paralysis was a very important part of their practice, and that they were aware of the value of the records that they were keeping. The Annual Reports 1760-1879 show the same results: of 3377 cases of paralysis due to lead admitted, 1533 (45.4%) were cured, and 3162 (93%) improved.

It might appear that this high success rate occurred because the patients were highly selected or the results of outcome were too optimistic but if one compares the cure rate of the paralyses due to lead with those of paralyses from other causes a marked difference is seen.

This is illustrated clearly in a broadsheet[14] printed in 1829 giving the aggregate of the patients of the Bath General Hospital between 1799 and 1828 and showing that the percentage of cures for all cases of paralyses was 20%. When this was broken down it showed that only 6% of the paralyses due to deformities of the spine and 11% of other paralyses not due to lead (often due to strokes) were cured. However 49% of the cases due to lead poisoning were discharged as cured. The variable cure rates indicate quite clearly that the doctors showed clinical judgement when assessing the outcome of the treatment of paralysis from different causes. The historical evidence suggests that Bath spa therapy was a very effective treatment of paralysis due to lead poisoning.

By using modern techniques it is possible to show how these high cure rates could have been achieved. Sitting in warm water up to the neck formed a vital part of the treatment in Bath; this immersion factor could have contributed to the cures claimed by the Bath Hospital. In the early 1970's Americans working on the N.A.S.A.[15] space programme found that it was possible to simulate the effects of weightlessness by sitting the would-be astronauts up to their necks in water at 35°C. With unlimited funds at his disposal, Murray Epstein was able to carry out extensive studies on the profound physiological effects of immersion on the human body. He found that during up-to-the-neck immersion the urinary excretion of water, sodium and calcium were markedly increased.

The external pressure exerted on a body immersed in water is directly proportional to the depth of the water at that point. Thus during immersion of the body in thermoneutral water whilst standing or sitting, there is a pressure gradient which increases with depth. Blood and some intercellular fluid is therefore expelled from the legs and the lower part of the body, this extra cellular fluid moving into the blood vessels in the thorax. This results in an increase in central blood volume of about 700 mls. in the right side of the circulation. As sensory receptors for blood volume appear to be situated in the right atrium this deceives the body, which reacts as though there had been an increase in total body fluid volume and not just a re-allocation of fluid.

The increase in right atrial pressure is thought to result in the release of certain hormones[16] into the circulation, so the body responds to this apparent increase in total fluid volume by greatly increasing not only the loss of water but also of sodium, potassium and calcium in an attempt to regain the equilibrium.

The cardiac output is increased by 50% at 35°C but there is no rise in blood pressure so the resistance of the peripheral circulation must be reduced by immersion in thermoneutral water. Immersion is also found to reduce the level of one of the naturally occurring adrenalin-like hormones, possibly one reason that bathing in warm water is found to be so relaxing.

These immersion studies indicate some of the mechanisms involved in the bathing element of spa therapy and which will be evoked by immersion in *any* water at 35°C.[17] They also suggests an explanation for some of the traditional contra-indications to spa therapy; recent cardiac infarction and pulmonary disease.

Could this immersion factor have contributed to the high cure rate for lead poisoning that was achieved in the Bath Hospital? The body handles lead and calcium in a similar way so we investigated the effects of immersion on the renal handling of lead.[18] The experiments were carried out in the Immersion Unit at the Bristol Royal Infirmary, when we were able to confirm Epstein's findings and to establish that urinary lead excretion is increased during immersion. Lead poisoning is very rare these days, but mild levels of intoxication are occasionally found in lead workers.

In Bristol, lead shot is manufactured in a traditional shot tower from where we were able to recruit some workers who volunteered to take part in our experiments. They were all-symptom free, with blood lead levels below the legal safety requirements. They therefore had a very much lower total body lead load than the patients who had been admitted to hospital with lead paralyses in the eighteenth century. Four lead workers volunteered to be immersed for three hours up to the neck in water at 35°C. They sat outside the tank for one hour before and after the immersion. Blood samples were taken before immersion and samples of urine collected hourly for the five hours of the experiment.

In essence we have measured urinary lead excretion basally and during a three hour immersion period. In all the subjects so far examined there was a large increase in the rate of urinary lead excretion during immersion. It was found to double in the first hour and quadruple during the second hour of immersion. The total amounts excreted during one three hour immersion period are small compared to the total body lead, which is predominantly tissue bound. However if these immersions were continued to the extent described in the hospital records (i.e. three times a week for 24 weeks) an appreciable proportion of the total body lead would be removed.

From these results we can suggest a mechanism through which the traditional Bath spa therapy could have operated. It is essential however that we do not disregard the other elements involved in the Bath spa treatment plan which included removal from the source of exposure and good food, nor disregard the beneficial effects of exercising in warm water or the therapeutic effects of drinking the mineral water. It contains 390 mgm of calcium per litre and iron in a soluble form, if drunk near to the source, as the amount of iron in solution is reduced after exposure to the oxygen in the air. Work done in north America[19] during the last decade has shown that calcium and iron deficiency increases the toxicity of that already in the body.[20] A recent U.S. report suggested giving calcium and iron supplements to deprived infants with raised blood lead levels.

So drinking the water could be helpful too. The eighteenth century doctors certainly thought it was an important part of the therapy. The effects of drinking the water is yet to be studied.

The founders of the Bath Hospital believed that by building up a bank of "indisputable evidence" it would eventually be possible to show that the Bath spa therapy could be recognised as an effective cure, not merely a pleasant experience. This paper is an attempt to justify their endeavours and to show that Bath spa therapy is a very effective treatment for chronic lead poisoning, the *Colica Pictonum*.

A Difcourfe of Naturall

B A T H E S,

And Minerall

VV A T E R S.

Wherein firft the originall of Fountaines
in generall, is declared.

Then the nature and differences of Minerals, with examples of particular Bathes from moft of them.

Next the generation of Minerals in the earth, from whence
both the actuall heat of Bathes, and their vertues
are proved to proceed.

Alfo by what meanes Minerall Waters are to bee examined and difcouered.

And laftly, of the nature and ufes of Bathes, but ef-
pecially of our Bathes at BATHE in Sommerfet-fhire.

The third Edition, much enlarged.

By ED. IORDEN, D^r. in Phyfick.

LONDON,
Printed by THO. HARPER. MDCXXXIII.

And are to be fold by *Michael Sparke* in Green Arbour.

33. Edward Jorden's Discourse on Mineral Waters — one of the earlier treatises on balneology.

ACKNOWLEDGEMENTS

This is a shortened version of a paper appearing in *The Medical History of Spas and Waters,* edited by R.S. Porter and W.F. Bynum Medical History Supplement number 10.

I thank Bath City Council, The Swainn Foundation and the Bristol Kidney Fund for their financial support. I acknowledge the encouragement and the assistance that I received from Dr A.H. Waldron with the urinary lead analysis and from Mr. C. Quinnell for access to the Bath Hospital records. I thank also Dr. P O'Hare, Dr. N. Millar, Professor P.A.Dieppe and Dr J Campbell McKenzie for their help and for permission to use the Immersion tank in the Bristol Royal Infirmary.

REFERENCES

1. Charlton Rice, *Three Tracts on Bath Water*, Bath 1774, Wm Taylor, 2nd Ed. Tract 2, (2) pp 77-9; pp 12-13, (Table)

2. Citois Francis, *De novo et Populari apud Pictones dolore colico bilioso diatriba*, Paris, 1639. Quoted by Eisinger Jos, "Lead and Wine Erbhard Glockel and the Colica Pictonum", *Medical History* 1982, **26;** pp 279-302.

3. Baker Sir Geo, An inquiry concerning the Cause of the Endemic Colic of Devonshire, *Trans Coll Phys,* June 29 1767
    An Historical account, i*bid,* July 21 1767
    Observations on the poison of Lead, *ibid,* Dec 11 1771

4. Defoe D, *A Tour through Great Britain*, London, Folio Soc, Vol 2 p 170

5. Peirce, Robert, *The History and Memoirs of The Bath*, London 1713, Henry Hammond.

6. *The London Practice of Physic*, London 1778, p 189

7. Wynter John, *Of Bathing in the Hot Baths at Bathe*, London 1728, James Leake, p 53

8. Pepys Samuel, *Diary*, 13th June 1668

9. Fiennes Celia, *The Journeys of Celia Fiennes*, edited C Morris, Cresset Press, p 18

10. *History of the Royal Mineral Water Hospital*, Bath 1888, p 20-1 12

11. Archives of the Royal National Hospital for Rheumatic Diseases Bath
    Minute Book for 1754; *Referral Register* 1751-8; *Annual Reports* 1741-1870

12. Falconer, Wm, *On the Bath Waters*, London, G Robinson, 1807, pp 62-3

13. Summers John, *A Short Account of the success of Warm Bathing in Paralytic Disorders*, London, C Hitch & L Hawes, 1751, pp 4-7

14. Hunt collection; Bath Central Reference Library, Vol 1, p 232

15.   Epstein M, "Renal effects of Head out immersion in man", *Physiol Rev*, 1978, **58:**(3): pp 529-81

16.   Anderson J V, Millar N, O'Hare J P, Mackenzie R J C, Corrall R J M, "Do circulating levels of atrial naturetic peptide (ANP) mediate the naturetic response to water immersion in man?" *Clin Sci*, 1985, **69;** p39

17.   O'Hare P, Heywood A, et al "Observations on the effects of immersion in Bath Spa water", *B.M.J.*, 1985; **291;** p 1747

18.   Heywood A, Waldron H A, O'Hare P, Dieppe P A, "Effect of immersion on Urinary lead Excretion", *Brit Journ Indust Med*, 1986; **43;** pp 713-5

19.   Mahaffey K, Goyer R, Haseman J K, "Dose response to lead ingestion in rats fed low dietary calcium", *J Lab Clin Med*, 1973; **82;** pp 92-100

20.   Barton J C, et al "Effects of iron on the absorption and retention of lead", *J Lab. Clin. Med.* **92** (4) pp 536-47

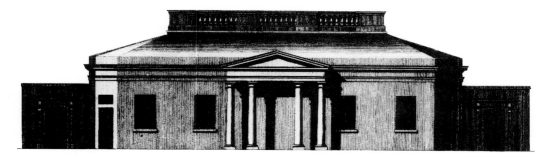

34. The Hot Bath at Bath, redesigned by John Wood the Younger. 1777.

FROM BALNEOLOGY TO PHYSIOTHERAPY: The development of physical treatment at Bath

Roger Rolls

There is nothing new about physiotherapy. It has been practised in one form or another since the earliest days of civilisation. Only the term is modern, coming into general use about half a century ago. Spas like Bath traditionally played an important role in the rehabilitation of physically handicapped patients. By looking at the way in which physical treatments have evolved at Bath, it is possible to identify some of the forerunners of modern physiotherapy.

The city has been a popular resort for crippled and physically disabled patients since the time of the Romans. As Smollett observed in his novel, *The Expedition of Humphrey Clinker*, published in 1772:

> One hobbled, another hopped, a third dragged his legs behind him like a wounded snake, a fourth was straddled betwixt a pair of long crutches like a mummy of a felon hanging in chains, a fifth was bent into a horizontal position like a mounted telescope and sixth was the bust of a man set up in a wheel machine.[1]

The principal salvation offered to these unfortunate characters lay in the hot mineral springs issuing forth in an incessant steamy stream from beneath the city.

The vogue for bathing has, rather like the water itself, ebbed and flowed over the centuries. During the Roman period, a fine suite of baths was constructed which has been re-excavated during the past two hundred years and forms one of the most important archaeological sites of this period in Britain. Though public baths were used as much for social purposes as for therapeutic, the Romans certainly advocated bathing as well as other forms of physical treatment. Galen recommended hot-air baths, followed by warm-water and massage for a number of diseases. Great store was put on the contrasting temperature of the various baths, so that patients moved from hot rooms to cold plunge baths or from vapour baths into warm water. Hot bathing was frequently followed by massage, or scraping of the skin with a *strigil*.[2] This was usually done by servants, some of whom became particularly adept at wielding these instruments and may have made their living at the baths by attending those bathers who were unaccompanied by their own servant.

There is very little documentary evidence of who used the baths and how at Bath during the mediaeval period though they were certainly being used therapeutically in the twelfth century for the author of the *Gesta Stephani* relates how diseased people from all over England came to wash away their infirmities in the healing waters.[3] Interest appears to have been re-awakened in the sixteenth century by the publication of two

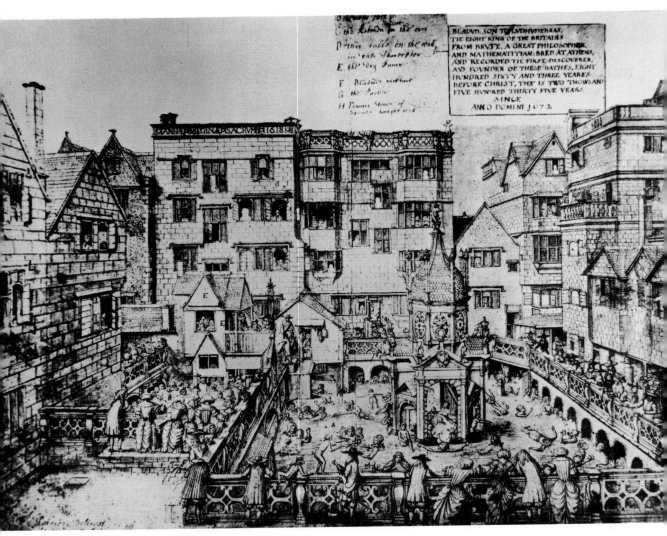

35. The Kings Bath in 1675, by Thomas Johnson. *(from an original in The British Museum).*

books on therapeutic bathing by Dr John Jones[4] and Dr William Turner.[5] Turner lamented the shabbiness of English baths when compared with those in Germany and Italy. In Turner's time there were at least three baths in use at Bath, the King's, Cross and Hot Baths. There was possibly a fourth which would have been within the precincts of the abbey before its dissolution, and is depicted on a sixteenth century plan of the city as the Mild Bath.[6]

Further publications began to appear on bathing, and more specifically on the Bath Water, and visits by several members of the Royal Family in the first half of the seventeenth century helped to popularise the town as an important medical centre. It was also the only British town with natural hot springs, though both Buxton and Bristol had tepid waters. Bath had also improved its facilities for bathers and they were now far ahead of any other British spa.

Nevertheless, hydrotherapy at this time was fairly unsophisticated as Thomas Johnson's view of the King's Bath in 1675 suggests. The structure in the centre, erected over the hot spring, was known as the *kitchen* on account of the high temperature of the water there and had a habit of gradually subsiding into the bottom of the bath on account of the continual erosion taking place at the spring head. The bathing looks quite unruly with both sexes in the water together, and many are totally naked. Children appear to clamber on the surrounding parapet and dogs, cats and other assorted creatures were, according to John Wood, often hurled over the side to the amusement of the onlookers and the annoyance of the bathers.[7] Despite this, a certain degree of order prevailed. From the mid sixteenth century onwards, each bath was supervised by a Bath Keeper who rented his bath from the city council which was the freehold owner of all the baths in the city following the Reformation. The Bath Keeper's business involved allocating duties to a number of lesser officials and seeing "that everything in the bath is done peacefully, quietly and modestly". The *Directores Balnei*, later called Bath Guides, were appointed by the city council. The Council Minutes in the late seventeenth century give the names of eight men and six women for the King's Bath and four men and four women for the other two baths.[8]

Their duties included the supply of linen to bathers, cleaning the baths once daily after the water was drained out and collecting mud and scum from the floor of the bath[7] which was retained for use as cataplasms (poultices) for treating painful joints and skin conditions. The *Directores Balnei* also accompanied the bathers into the water, helping them into the bath if they were too disabled. Finally, in the eighteenth century, they were responsible for recording the temperature of the water and regulating it to between 98°F and 100°F [9] Ned Ward, a hack writer visiting Bath at the end of the seventeenth century observed that there were a score or two of guides at work who "by their scorbutic carcasses and lackered hides, (one) would think they had laid pickling a century of years in the Stygian Lake."[10]   Bathers employed "those infernal emissaries" to support their limbs or "scrub their putrifying carcasses like racehorses."[10]

Scrubbing the skin seems to have been the most common adjunct to bathing. Whereas the Romans used the strigil on the skin, the *Directores Balnei* favoured the use of the flesh-brush. In the early ledger and incidental book belonging to the Bath General Hospital, now the Royal National Hospital for Rheumatic Diseases, there are frequent orders for flesh-brushes.[11] These were rubbed up and down paralytic or rheumatic limbs to stimulate the skin circulation, much for the same reason that birch twigs are now wielded in sauna baths. Curiously, the various treatises on the Bath Waters published in the seventeenth and eighteenth centuries make little mention of this early form of massage.

Though the hospital employed its own Bath Guides in the eighteenth century, much of the scrubbing appears to have been done by the nurses - perhaps the origin of the somewhat derogatory expression of scrubber. As late as 1820, Dr Edward Barlow, a physician at the Mineral Water Hospital, lamented that the standard of nursing was so low that the nursing staff could not even manage to perform shampooing, the term then used for this particular type of rubbing. From the mid- nineteenth century, the hospital took on a specialised nurse known as a rubber.[12]

Another reference to rubbing comes in the *New Bath Guide* of 1788, written by the poet Christopher Anstey:

> And of all the fine sights I have seen, my dear mother,
> I never expect to behold such another:
> How the ladies did giggle and set up their clacks
> All the while an old woman was rubbing their backs.[13]

The term rubber seems to have been dropped at Bath in favour of the grander-sounding *masseur* around 1890, though there was a short period during which the Mineral Water Hospital employed both a rubber and a masseur. The adoption of the French terminology coincides with the development of more sophisticated hydrotherapy facilities which took place in the late nineteenth century. Many of the so-called wet masseurs were trained in foreign spas. During the First World War, the hospital employed several blind ex-servicemen as masseurs. The blind seem to have had some particular talent for this sort of treatment.

For years, indeed for centuries, the most sophisticated technological innovation which Bath had been able to offer was a number of hand pumps, in and near the baths, which were used to direct strong jets of mineral water onto particular parts of the body. The pumps were originally operated by the Bath Guides who received extra payment for their labours which could sometimes involve giving as many as 2000 strokes of the pump to a patient. The pumps were installed in the early seventeenth century and largely displaced the earlier practice of bucketing whereby two guides tipped bucketfuls of hot mineral water over the patients affected parts,[5] or allowed the water to run out of a hole in the floor of the bucket.

Rumblings of discontent over the primitive state of the baths were expressed in the mid-eighteenth century by a surgeon, Archibald Cleland, who was later expelled from his honorary post at the hospital on account of professional misconduct. Cleland submitted plans to the Mayor of Bath, Ralph Allen, in 1739, in which he proposed that the council should build a suite of hot and cold baths offering privacy and cover from the inclemencies of the British climate.[14] His plans were never adopted though a more modern suite of private baths was developed about twenty years later on land owned by the Duke of Kingston.

Major developments took place in the nineteenth century with the arrival of a mind-boggling assortment of hydro-mechanical and hydro-pneumatic gadgets, most of which took their names from various continental Spas:- the Plombière Douche - a polite way of describing an enema of mineral water; The Neuheim Sprudel Bad, a sort of jacuzzi which, with a bevy of attractive therapists on hand, was guaranteed to take the mind off virtually any ailment; and the Aix Douche, no more really than the traditional "dry pump" except that the water was delivered from the efforts of a steam engine rather than a person. Another version of this involved alternative hot and cold douches, known rather euphemistically as a Scotch Douche. This was used to "tone up" the circulatory and nervous systems. Needle baths also served this function, the fine jets of water providing a strong physical stimulus on the skin, particularly when the temperature was alternated between hot and cold.

Massage was frequently combined with mineral water therapies. The Vichy apparatus was used as a way of administering wet massage, the attendants clad in large unwieldy rubber aprons worn somewhat incongruously over bathing costumes.

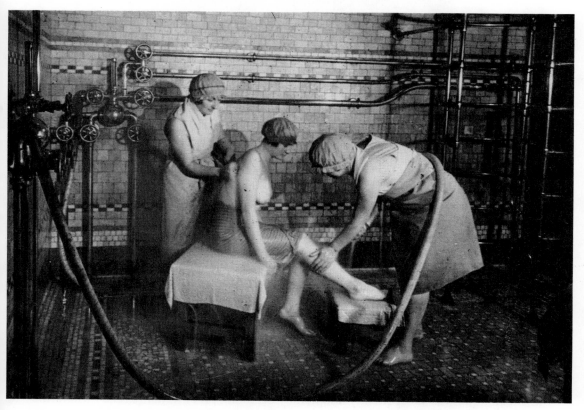

36. Wet massage. The patient receives combined treatment from an Aix douche and a flesh brush, held by the lady on the left. Bath Spa. Early 20th century.

Though hydrotherapy was the principal form of physical treatment practised at Bath, there appears to have been an early, if somewhat cautious, interest in electrotherapy. Dr Edward Harington (1696-1757) made some experiments on paralytic patients admitted to the Bath Hospital just prior to his death in 1757 but was unimpressed by his results. Dr Rice Charleton (1723-1789), in a publication in 1774[15] expressed considerable doubt over the usefulness of electricity, possibly because it was being favoured by the quack doctor, James Graham, who was practising in the area at that time.

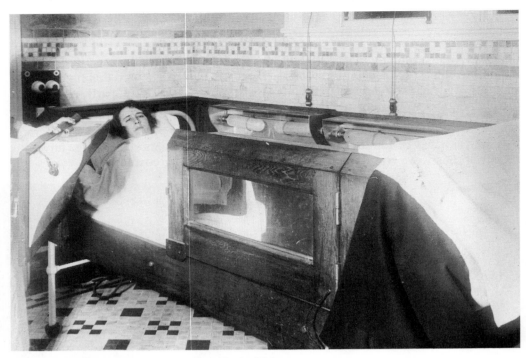

37.　An electric light bath. Bath Spa. Early 20th century.

Graham, besides advocating cold earth and warm mud bathing was keen to promote magnetism and electricity as therapeutic tools.[16] Mud bathing was certainly popular at various times during the Spa's history though it was only Graham who adopted a positively voyeuristic approach to treatment. Peirce mentions its use at the end of the seventeenth century. "In many cases this Mudd is apply'd by way of a Cataplasm, chiefly in hard white swellings, and contractions of the limbs (where it may be conveniently apply'd) or where a callous or slimy matter is wedg'd into a part or joynt, or when wind distends it and so causes a painful swelling and hinders a due and ready motion of that Limb."[17] Until 1976, when the Spa was closed, mud packs were made from fullers' earth, mined on the southern slopes of the city, and hot mineral water.

Graham had also suggested using electricity applied through the medium of baths and this technique was subsequently adopted by orthodox practitioners in the form of the four-cell Schnee bath.

With the arrival of mains electricity, the scope for gadgets was greatly enlarged and at the turn of the century, the Spa department at Bath proudly developed an electrical room, complete with a electric couch on which an unsuspecting patient could lie and be given a stealthful shock or two through conductors hidden in the upholstery. The Mineral Water Hospital, anxious to develop its capacity for electrotherapists, set up its own electrical department in 1913. Once again, it was nurses who took over the role of electrotherapist.

There is a certain parallel to be seen between mineral water with its invisible healing powers and electricity, a mysterious and powerful flux capable of generating heat and other radiant forms of energy. Perhaps this accounted for the obsession of incarcerating patients in boxes where the elusive power could be concentrated and retained. In the case of mineral water, the patient was placed in a wooden box, sealed up as effectively as was possible while still retaining the option for respiration to continue. Wooden boxes were later replaced by metal cabinets but the principle was the same.

In the case of electricity, the hidden forces could be concentrated in a similar manner, either in the form of the electric light bath, or in a Greville Electric Bath, a large cylinder not unlike an iron lung in which the patient could be baked like a roast chicken with temperatures exceeding 300°F.

During the first part of the present century, massage and electrotherapy ran along parallel, but separate, courses. It was in spas where they were drawn together, albeit rather tenuously and at times perhaps even dangerously through the medium of water. The final fusion of electrotherapist with masseur has led to the modern physiotherapist, a fusion which was fostered by the peculiar situation which obtained in spas. Hydrotherapy, untrammelled by its previous association with mineral content and quintessential principles of its medium, is still very much a part of the physiotherapist's armamentarium in this city.

In summary, the physiotherapist, at least in the spa town, seems to have evolved from a mixed ancestry. She can claim a direct descent from the *Directores Balnei* of the seventeenth century but also has connections with nurses, quacks and blind ex-servicemen.

38. A turbine bath.

39. A patient about to enter a steam cabinet.

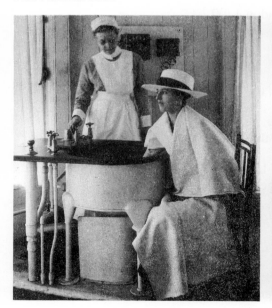

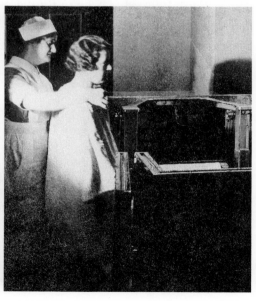

REFERENCES

1.   Smollett T, *The Expedition of Humphrey Clinker*, London 1771

2.   Ryley Scott, George, *The story of baths and bathing*, Laurie, London 1939, p 46

3.   *Gesta Stephani*, 2nd edn, ed and trans by Potter K R, 1976

4.   Jones J, *The Bathes of Bathes Ayde*, London 1572

5.   Turner W, *A Book of the Natures and Properties of the Baths of England*, Arnold Birkman, Colen [Cologne] 1562

6.   Plan of Bath by William Smith in the British Museum, 1588, British Library, Sloane MS 2596

7.   Wood J, *An Essay Towards a Description of Bath*, 1749, reprinted in 1969 by Kingsmead Press, Bath

8.   James P R, *The Baths of Bath in the sixteenth and early seventeenth centuries*, Arrowsmith, Bristol 1938

9.   Minute Book 1783 (in possession of the Royal National Hospital for Rheumatic Diseases, Bath)

10.   Ward, Edward, *A Step to Bath*, London 1700

11.   see Rolls R, *The Hospital of the Nation*, Bird Publications, Bath 1988, pp 55 and 129

12.   Minute Book, 1852 (in possession of the Royal National Hospital for Rheumatic Diseases, Bath)

13.   Anstey C, *The New Bath Guide*, 13th ed 1788, p 46

14.   Cleland A, *An Appeal to the Public*, London 1743, MSS notes by Cleland in the front of the copy held by Cambridge University Library

15.   Charleton R, *Three Tracts on the Bath Waters*, Bath 1774

16.   Graham J, *A New, Plain and Rational Treatise on the true nature and uses of the Bath Waters*, Bath 1789

17.   Peirce, Robert, *The History and Memoirs of the Bath*, London 1713, p 244

MEDICAL APPRENTICES IN EIGHTEENTH CENTURY ENGLAND

Joan Lane

As an institution apprenticeship has had a bad press. At the poorest end of the employment spectrum the factory child and climbing boy are heart-rending, while the most prosperous occupations such as medicine and law prefer not to recall their apprenticed origins. Yet for the surgeon-apothecary in eighteenth century England training by apprenticeship was universal, valued and a considerable financial investment. From the early mediaeval period apprenticeship was the legally enforced means of technical training for entry into a wide range of occupations; Campbell cited over 300 in London in 1747 and these increased during the century.[1] Irrespective of occupational standing, certain factors were common to all crafts and trades, including medicine: money (the premium) was paid to the master, in whose home the apprentice lived for a fixed period of time (the term), a written agreement (the indenture) was signed, since an oral arrangement was not legally binding, and the master was to teach and board the child in exchange for the apprentice's labour. From one occupation to another there were, obviously, variations, with great differences between, for example, a prosperous cabinet maker, gunsmith or saddler and a poor carpenter, tailor or shoemaker. At the very top of the pyramid were the great London traders, dealing in valuable raw materials, with warehouses, large stocks or risk capital; to such masters boys took huge premiums, £1000 to a silk broker in 1783[2] or £1075 to a Levant merchant.[3] Even gentlemen's younger sons, from old-established families, by the eighteenth century were becoming apprentices and some masters seem to have taken well-bred boys with lower premiums, presumably for the cachet of having them in a business or practice, for where one youthful gentleman went, other parents would think it proper to place their sons. Many instances exist of bequests made to enable a child to be apprenticed with a good premium if his father were to die; indeed, the numbers of widows binding boys as apprentices is quite striking at this period.

The premium in the monetarist eighteenth century is the surest yardstick of occupational status left to us after two hundred years and the range of medical premiums illuminates the profession's enhanced status, new variety of responsibilities, increased skills and upward social mobility in Georgian England. It is possible to explain these changes in one way and argue that the separation of the surgeons from the barbers in 1745 made medical careers more socially acceptable, removing practitioners from the humble connotations of the barbers' craft, but this is a simplistic explanation that ignores the wider aspects of medical practice and contemporary perceptions of status. Without the separation of the two occupations, it seems likely that surgeons would have remained in the apothecaries' category in the eighteenth century and certainly not have attained the eminence of the famous surgical practitioners in Georgian England. Apart from these considerations, external factors in society combined to enhance the surgeon's position.
In a consumerist and affluent age, patients expected more medical attention of an

increasingly sophisticated nature than was available in the early 1700s; patients had more disposable income, were willing to spend it on services, even luxuries, rather than, as formerly, simply on the basic essentials of life. An expanding population, with increased expectation of life by the mid years of the century, a prosperous, often booming economy as England's colonies thrived and above all decades of relative domestic peace under the Hanoverians, all assisted a burgeoning medical profession. Wider education and literacy in addition meant that the population at large was better informed about medicine in the widest sense and people's expectations were raised. In a rational, doubting age, medicine was perceived more as an exercise of science than as questioning the will of God.

Contemporary provincial newspapers (of which there were over thirty by the 1750s) always contained a wide range of medical items, cases treated, epidemics feared, hospitals opened, interesting operations performed. Practitioners themselves were a constant source of interest, to judge from the frequency with which their activities were reported; personal events, (such as marriages and deaths), thefts or physical violence they suffered, institutional appointments, changes of surgery premises, all appeared regularly in the eighteenth century press. Practitioners, as well as a wide range of quacks, used the press to advertise their services and it is in this expanding, materialist period that medical apprenticeships must be seen as a chance for recently prosperous boys to enter an occupation above their fathers', but also a career newly suitable for youths of professional or even gentry origins.

For entry into medicine in the eighteenth century, however, a money yardstick was important; a master expected a premium with his apprentice to cover the youth's board, lodging and tuition during a seven or, less often, a five year term, as well as compensate for the patients he might offend, the raw materials he might spoil or the various errors he might make. Certain factors determined the premium in medicine as in other occupations; the master's status, the prospects of future employment and earning capacity, the parents' willingness to pay the required sum, the master's personal eagerness to have or avoid a particular apprentice. A medical family, a gentry or *nouveau riche* background, for instance, might be differently assessed by the intending master and the premium adjusted accordingly. The slow inflation of the period meant that premiums changed for other reasons; many masters took premiums little different from their own a decade or more earlier, but external factors, such as a hospital, a great house, cathedral or prosperous spa in the area, could raise premiums quite substantially. London masters, even if not famous, regularly took larger sums as premiums in all occupations.

A group of boys bound to Northampton masters in the eighteenth century emphasises the differences a hospital post could make to a master's status and hence to his premiums. In 1743 Charles Lyon was appointed to the new hospital there; in 1732 he had taken £42 with an apprentice, but in 1742 the premium was £60 and ten years later he received £100, in each case for a seven year term, and the youths were allowed to attend the hospital, watch and assist at operations. Lyon himself had been indentured in 1714 with £48.⁴ A similar situation existed at Birmingham, where the infirmary opened in 1779. Thomas Tomlinson had worked in Birmingham from 1760, when he was appointed as workhouse surgeon after having trained in London at St George's under Caesar Hawkins, David Middleton and William Bromfield.⁵ His first two apprentices paid £60 and £80 respectively; his third, in 1777, when it was apparent that the hospital could not be much longer delayed, brought £105. However, after the infirmary opened in 1779 Tomlinson's last two apprentices paid £105 and £150 each in 1780 and 1782.⁶ In counties without hospitals a different scale of premiums is apparent, as are the sums paid to masters who might never, in a remote country area, have more than an immediate locality as their practice. George Crabbe exemplifies the poorer medical apprentice, obliged to sleep and share his social life with the farm boy. A direct contrast can be seen in Wiltshire between rural and urban medical apprentices; in Pewsey a country surgeon took £35 with a boy, whereas in Salisbury sums of between £140 and £210 were paid.⁷ In London in 1747 Campbell advised parents to pay a premium of £20 to £200 to an apothecary and from £20 to £100 to a surgeon,⁸ but almost as he wrote, John Harrison at the London Hospital was able to command premiums of £250 and £367.⁹ In the counties of Surrey, Sussex, Warwickshire and Wiltshire, during the half century from 1710 to 1760, 132 premiums from £20 to 80 guineas were paid, with £60 or £63 most commonly recorded (25.7 per cent).¹⁰ Following the precept that premiums were, in practice, what the master could extract from a boy's parents, the exact sum required was virtually never mentioned when vacant apprenticeships were advertised in the press. Some masters stated that the premium would be "reasonable" or "substantial", but all emphasised that the boy would have a "good place" and live as family, stressing the qualities required of the applicant, who was expected to be sober, of good family, well educated and often also well recommended.

How masters and apprentices found each other in the eighteenth century largely depended on the status of the occupation. The most prosperous masters did not need to advertise vacancies for youths and the poorest men relied on word of mouth, but a wide range of occupations, including medicine, increasingly used press advertisements to find apprentices. Since some 7.5 million newspapers were sold in 1750 and almost double by 1780¹¹ advertising was a particularly effective way of a master's reaching intending apprentices and their parents, as well as announcing his services to the readership, even if in a discreet manner:

> Wanted: A Sober, Careful Young Man, of good Family, to serve as an Apprentice to an Apothecary, Surgeon and Man Midwife; if he has served some time to the Business he will be full as well approv'd of. Anyone well recommended, by directing to J B at the Crown, Lichfield St, Birmingham, will meet with an undeniable Place.¹²

With improved communications, especially by road, greater literacy, a larger population and enhanced medical career opportunities, more boys travelled further to find masters by the mid eighteenth century, and London remained a magnet for apprentices whose parents could afford the larger premiums charged there. However, apprentices in the provinces, if bound to men of good and extensive practice, could receive a broad and comprehensive medical training even if not attached to county hospitals. Thus in Coventry, where Bradford Wilmer was a surgeon-apothecary, his four apprentices saw a wide range of cases in the later eighteenth century. The son of a cleric and nephew of a Buckinghamshire apothecary, Wilmer was taught by John Hunter, with whom he remained in correspondence, as well as by Sharpe, and was one of a four-man practice for forty years. He served four parishes as poor law surgeon, did dissections and second opinions, especially difficult deliveries, and kept a notebook of his cases, including amputations and couching. He was an expert witness in several murder trials, such as the laurel-water murder of Sir Theodosius Boughton, and had wide scientific interests. He took four apprentices in the years 1773-95, with premiums of £130 to £210,[13] and, treating local patients from the aristocracy to the poor, boys bound to such a man would have had a very wide training, except for hospital work. Wilmer was awarded an MD by his monumental mason, but was essentially the skilled and experienced apprenticed man, of high repute in his locality and certainly capable of teaching his four apprentices individually and to a high level.

The social origins of surgeon-apothecaries' apprentices rose during the eighteenth century; from four English counties in the period 1710-60, 17 medical apprentices listed in the London registers were fatherless (whose mothers paid premiums from 45 to 100 guineas), seven fathers were gentlemen, five were clerics, five large traders and three were medical practitioners. Only two were of fairly humble origins, described as a blacksmith and gate-keeper, but able to pay £50 premiums. At a later period in Coventry, of the eleven boys recorded, two were their masters' sons and two were orphans, while a farmer, cleric, button manufacturer, currier and carrier were also given as parents. Surgeons' prosperity may be measured in the occupations to which they bound their own sons; in Coventry their sons were indentured to substantial manufacturers but the practitioner's precarious hold on status and security is seen when a boy's father died, so that, for example, a Coventry surgeon's orphan son was bound to a humble watchmaker.[14] In medical families, although apprenticeship was regularly recorded, premiums were not paid. Some families, such as the Brees, the Kimbells and the Welchmans, all in Warwickshire, span two or three centuries, for not only the great London practitioners, such as the Hawkins family, formed "dynastic chains" in medicine. Surgeons only rarely broke the law regulating the numbers of apprentices a man might take at any one time; generally a single youth was all a master trained, although increasingly during the eighteenth century surgeon-apothecaries would take new boys into a practice as older ones were nearing the end of the term. Such an overlap added to the role-models an apprentice might see, alongside his master and perhaps a newly qualified assistant.

Medical apprentices were generally well-treated, not runaways or criminals and virtually never abandoned because of their masters' bankruptcy. Their duties, however, and position within the host household were the lowliest; medical apprentices were obliged to undertake the most menial tasks, washing and labelling bottles, rolling pills, sweeping floors and delivering medicine to patients. Later they were allowed to undertake tooth extraction, blood letting and helping with the accounts. Their hours of work were uncertain and they might expect only the great public holidays (Christmas, Easter and Whitsun); essentially they served patients' requirements, and Richard Kay recorded the long hours both he and his father worked, especially during a fever epidemic of 1757.[15] Medical instruction was essentially practical, and Henry Jephson, apprenticed to a Nottinghamshire parish surgeon, wrote home in delight that he had been permitted to accompany his master on his rounds:

> I can with just pleasure add that he behaved like a Gent and has promised to let me visit them alone. I assure you it has happened exactly right in my last year, as I can visit them more than I did before, indeed he advised me to pay attention to the various diseases I see, and you may depend upon my taking it.[16]

The increase in the number of medical practitioners in the eighteenth century is a striking one. Until 1779 no national medical register existed and Samuel Foart Simmon's first version was greatly improved in the third edition of 1783. However, in individual communities, with trade directories and other listings, it is possible to see how their numbers expanded. Birmingham provides a good example of the growth of medical practice and the ratio of practitioners to patients at different periods:

Date	Practitioners (omitting MDs)	Population	Ratio
1767	20[17]	c.40,000[18]	1:2000
1785	21[19]	52,250[20]	1:2500
1793	39[21]	+60,000[22]	1:1600
1818	45[23]	85,416[24]	1:1900
1828	65[25]	110,914[26]	1:1700

A similar picture can be seen in other communities, even allowing for the scarcity of census type statistics before 1801 and the major problem of listing practitioners before the 1779-83 *Medical Registers* were published. Surgeons and apothecaries were always included in late eighteenth century trade directories, and there are medical entries for the larger towns in *The Universal British Directory* (1791-98). Birmingham, fortunately, was surveyed earlier for this purpose than any other provincial town, and has practitioners listed for 1767 and 1771; a publication as early as 1752 appears not to have survived. In addition, the phenomenal rise in its population encouraged comment long before government censuses were taken.

However, professional expansion really depends on an increased range of medical tasks and career opportunities, all bringing new sources of income. The majority of these appointments were institutional or public posts, many with annual salaries or contract fees, and for the practitioner such an arrangement was beneficial. Institutions paid at regular intervals, monthly, quarterly or annually, or on a *per capita* basis (for mass inoculation sessions or inspecting militia men and pauper factory apprentices, for example). Poor law work also expanded greatly in the eighteenth century, with unprecedented expenditure, medical fees being a regular commitment out of the parish rate. Overseers sought unavailingly to limit costs and increasingly in urban and larger rural parishes they negotiated a medical contract enabling them to forecast expenditure.

Public and institutional appointments were the most expanding area of medical practice in the eighteenth century, however. The most prestigious public office for a practitioner, and after 1752 relatively well paid, was that of Coroner. Coroners' bills were settled by the Justices, at Quarter Sessions, for fees and travelling claims submitted. The new Act (25 Geo. II, c 29) allowed coroners £1 for every inquest conducted outside a gaol and 9d a mile for journeys to inspect a body. The coroner's vouchers added considerably to a county's expenses after 1752. For example, in Hertfordshire Samuel Atkinson, who served for over thirty years, regularly received sums totalling £30 to £60 a year and, with fees and travel rates unchanged, his duties and income obviously expanded considerably. The hazards of his office, however, are apparent; in the winter of 1758-9 gaol fever was a danger to the coroner's jury when they went "to view the dead bodies" and in 1773 the prisoners were bought clean clothes to "make them clean and free from infection for their Trials".[27] In counties as different as Wiltshire[28] and Warwickshire a similar range of coroners' fees was paid.[29] Some large cities, such as Coventry and Birmingham, also had their own appointees; thus in 1764-5, for example, the Birmingham coroner was paid £18 7s 6d for attending 15 investigations and travelling 86 miles.[30] How the office was valued may be judged from the competition in medical and legal circles to fill a vacancy.

Far more opportunities for medical practitioners were available lower down the professional scale in the eighteenth century, which witnessed a substantial growth in gaol, bridewell, workhouse, asylum, dispensary and hospital posts throughout the provinces. Largely as a result of contemporary philosophy towards deviants, criminals and the deserving poor, if only because their numbers, as part of the total population expansion, grew perceptibly, institutions for different categories were established at an increasing rate as the century progressed. Penal institutions were always served by a surgeon or apothecary, also paid by Quarter Sessions, and their *per capita* fees were, after c 1750, commuted into an annual contract sum. Thus, in Hertfordshire, Richard Cutler received £10 a year in the 1760s, which doubled in the next decade, whereas in the 1750s his predecessors had been paid various sums for medicines and attention;[31] in Warwickshire the gaol surgeon-apothecary, George Weale, switched to an annual payment of £20 in 1764. He was appointed in 1755 and for a decade was paid £30 or more a year, including special extra sums for treating smallpox in the gaol in 1758 and 1762. It may have been competition that made him agree to accept a contract at £20 p.a.,[32] but he obviously valued the post because when, in 1777 he took his son, Edward, as a partner, the partnership deed specified that the gaol appointment was a personal not a practice one, and that he would keep the income.[33] Workhouses were a further source of employment for the surgeon-apothecary in the eighteenth century.   At Birmingham, for example, the three workhouse surgeons each received £18 a year until 1741, when it increased to £25 a year;[34] one of these men was Edward Audley, who commanded a premium of £100 in 1761 with his apprentice,[35] John Derrington, who himself later became a poor law surgeon in Edgbaston parish. There were more workhouses in the English counties in the eighteenth century than has generally been presumed; 29 in Warwickshire by 1776 with 1819 inhabitants,[36] for example, and with surgeons' salaries in the £50 range.

Lunatic asylums became an expanding area of medical practice in the eighteenth century but they are difficult to assess as a source of income to the practitioner for lack of records. However, at a weekly charge of a guinea, excluding linen and laundry,[37] with only ten inmates an asylum keeper's steady income was £540 a year; many patients were inmates for decades and most asylums admitted far more patients than this. Hospitals and dispensaries are difficult to judge as a source of expanding medical employment in the eighteenth century, as hospital appointments, except the house apothecary and men in military and naval establishments, were honorary, unpaid posts.   Undeniably, however, hospital appointees were able to charge enhanced premiums and their apprentices secured a training that often enabled them in turn to climb the professional ladder. However, it was only after 1740 that hospitals were founded outside London in numbers that made training places and posts available. By 1783 there were twenty-six provincial hospitals in existence, but seventeen English counties had no infirmary while other areas (Lancashire, Somerset and Yorkshire) had two or three each. These hospitals actually provided posts for 76 physicians and 86 surgeons, of whom only the two at Staffordshire were paid (£30 p a each),[38] but a further fifteen apothecaries held residential hospital posts as full time appointments, often the first career step for some young practitioners. Contemporary interest in the founding of hospitals was such that new infirmaries were always mentioned in the press, their subscriptions, premises and appointments regularly reported, as were their changes of staff and patient success rates.

Dispensaries were in every respect less prestigious, although probably influencing the health of more inhabitants than the county infirmaries of the period. By 1783 there were eight dispensaries established quite randomly in the provinces, all founded in the last decade, each with two or three practitioners in attendance.[39] They provided excellent training prospects for the apprentice, since many of them claimed very large numbers of patients attending, and, by the nineteenth century, were to offer extended employment opportunities to young practitioners.

A further aspect of institutional medical care in the eighteenth century, regrettably often regarded as a nineteenth century phenomenon, was the cover and attention provided by the Friendly Societies, of which there were an enormous number. Since they were primarily mutual benefit, insurance, accident and burial organisations, rather than embryonic trades unions, they all needed medical advice for their members who wished to benefit, and especially when any claims were contested. The society officers sought medical advice, with appropriate sick notes and paid practitioners for their attention. Some of the societies' rules specifically excluded members and claims on medical grounds. For example, men in some dangerous trades, especially mining and metal working, might not join, nor might members seek benefit if their injuries were sustained from fighting, football, wrestling or violence, while those with venereal diseases were also excluded. Medical practitioners were paid by the friendly societies at negotiated rates, of which those for a Lichfield society, which began in 1770, are typical. The surgeon-apothecary was paid 1s 6d for each member a year in the city limits and 2s 6d for those beyond this area to cover a maximum of two house visits a week. This particular society did not limit its membership numbers and thus the surgeon's related income.[40] Friendly Society medical certificates of injury or illness, although a very rare category of archive for the eighteenth century, have occasionally survived as a further aspect of expanding professional duties. There were other aspects of practice, new medications, treatments (such as electric and hydrotherapy), surgery and techniques, of which inoculation was the most profitable, that expanded medicine after c1750 to an unprecedented degree, creating professional opportunities unimagined by the barber-surgeon earlier in the century. Although specialisms are generally seen as a nineteenth century development, their origins can be discerned in Georgian England, especially in obstetrics, ophthalmology and forensic medicine. The continuous rise in population, linked with a booming economy and society's greatly increased expectations of material comforts in daily life, all coincided to make opportunities for the medical profession to be expansionist as never before. Many men were skilled and fortunate, able to take advantage of the new circumstances offered by Georgian society; a contemporary commented that the surgeon should be both ingenious and humane, but could attain "inward satisfaction and all the external blessings of wealth", [41] a goal for many apprentices to attain.

The merits of apprenticeship were considerable; the master-boy relationship enabled the youth to learn a life-style alongside occupational skills. He discovered how to run a practice as a business, especially if he were not from a medical family, planning visits, keeping records, buying drugs and equipment, sending bills, managing patients and judging the urgency of calls. The value of apprenticeship may best be seen in personal terms, the importance an apprentice attached to the name of the man with whom he had served his time, usually cited in advertisements, and the master's own regard for his former apprentices, to judge from the frequency with which bequests were made to them. Its drawbacks were its conservatism, its lack of both specialist teaching and a curriculum; the master's ability to instruct was never assessed. However, its undoubted advantages produced by the later eighteenth and early nineteenth century a range of distinguished and innovative English practitioners. In 1747 Campbell appositely summarised a surgeon's career in advising intending apprentices:

An ingenious Surgeon, let him be cast on any Corner of the Earth, with but his Case of Instruments in his Pocket, he may live where most other Professions would starve.[42]

REFERENCES

1. R Campbell, *The London Tradesman*, London, 1747, pp 331-40

2. Alfred Plummer, *The London Weavers' Company, 1600-1970*, London, 1972, p 76

3. J G L Burnby, *Apprenticeship Records*, British Society for the History of Pharmacy, 1977, **I,** 4, p 151

4. F F Waddy, *A History of Northampton General Hospital, 1743-1948*, Northampton, 1974, pp 19-20

5. T Tomlinson, *Medical Miscellany*, Birmingham, 1769

6. P J Wallis, R V Wallis and T D Whittet, *Eighteenth Century Medics*, Newcastle-upon-Tyne University, 1985, pp 1115-6

7. Christabel Dale (ed), *Wiltshire Apprentices and their Masters, 1710-60*, Devizes, 1981, Wiltshire Record Society, XVII

8. Campbell, op cit, pp 331, 339

9. A E Clark-Kennedy, *London Pride, the Story of a London Voluntary Hospital*, London, 1979

10. Joan Lane, "The Role of Apprenticeship in eighteenth century Medical Education" in W F Bynum and Roy Porter (eds), *William Hunter and the Eighteenth Century Medical World*, C U P, 1985, p 70

11. Jeremy Black, *The English Press in the Eighteenth Century*, London, 1987, p 290

12. *Aris's Birmingham Gazette*, 23 December 1754

13. Wallis, op cit, p 1224

14. Joan Lane (ed), *Coventry Apprentices and their Masters, 1781-1806*, Oxford, 1983, Dugdale Society, XXXIII

15. W Brockbank and F Kenworthy (eds), *The Diary of Richard Kay of Baldingstone, 1716-51*, 1968, Chetham Society, XVI, 3rd series

16. Warwick County Record Office, Z574

17. *Sketchley's Birmingham, Wolverhampton and Walsall Directory*, Birmingham, 1767, pp 2-3

18. Tomlinson, op cit, p 204

19. Samuel Foart Simmons, *The Medical Register for the Year 1783*, London, p 114

20. *Victoria History of the County of Warwick*, Oxford, 1964, VIII, p 8

21. *The Universal Trade Directory*, London, 1791-8, pp 207-8

22.   Ibid, p 202

23.   *Wrighton's Directory of Birmingham*, 1818 (medical names extracted)

24.   *V C H*, II, p 191 (census figures for 1821)

25.   *Pigot's Directory of Warwickshire*, 1828, p 805

26.   *V C H*, II, p 191 (census figures for 1831)

27.   W le Hardy (ed), *Hertfordshire County Records*, Hertford, 1935, VIII

28.   R F Hunnisett (ed), *Wiltshire Coroners' Bills, 1752-96*, Devizes, 1981, Wiltshire Record Society, XXXVI

29.   Warwick County Record Office, QS 39/5, 6, 7

30.   Ibid, QS 35A/2

31.   le Hardy, op cit

32.   Warwick County Record Office, QS 39/5, 6, 7

33.   Ibid, CR 1596/Box 90

34.   Birmingham Reference Library, 3870937

35.   Wallis, op cit, p 37

36.   Abstract of the Returns made by the Overseers of the Poor, 1777, pp 181-5

37.   Warwick County Record Office, CR 556/691

38.   *Med Reg, 1793*, op cit, and Joan Lane, "Medical Practitioners of Provincial England in 1783", *Medical History*, 1984, **28,** pp 353-71

39.   Ibid

40.   Lichfield Joint Record Office, D77/18/9

41.   Joseph Collyer, *The Parent's and Guardian's Directory*, London, 1761, p 270

42.   Campbell, op cit, p 57

EIGHTEENTH CENTURY MEDICS — the PHIBB Collective Biography

Peter and Ruth Wallis

The conception of the currently published work, *Eighteenth Century Medics,* came with the formation of the Book Subscription Lists Project in 1972, and its claim that book subscription lists were a largely unused but important historical record of significance in every aspect of British social history[1]. Medical history was clearly one of these significant fields, as many medical subscribers were identified, often by MD or surgeon/apothecary. This realisation was indicated concretely by the preparation, at an early stage of the work and at short notice, for the 1974 Cambridge Conference of the British Society for the History of Pharmacy of *A preliminary guide to apothecaries in book subscription lists*[2] (the general term "apothecaries" was interpreted to include also chemists, distillers, druggists and surgeons). Although based on less than a hundred lists and giving 322 names from about a hundred different towns, this preliminary essay was very encouraging - the baby was thriving. A major problem for the Project was seen as the identification of the apothecaries, so it was a natural next step to link up with Dr Whittet's valuable, wide-ranging work in preparing *A directory of provincial apothecaries*, announced in 1970. Apart from Society of Apothecaries and other national records, his collection included material from many provincial centres, often provided by local individual and institutional correspondents, but unfortunately his death prevents a contribution to the new edition.

It had soon been realised that a most invaluable and massive source was the Public Record Office Inland Revenue (medical) apprenticeship records[3] (made available by Dr Burnby), which could be supplemented by details of Bishops' Licences (held by the Wellcome Library)[4] and PHIBB's extensive files of subscription lists entered on the main-frame computer at Newcastle University. The combination of these three sources in an integrated alphabetical sequence of names was the backbone of the first edition[5], an impossible task without computers.

Each apprenticeship record contains the names of apprentice (A) and master (M) and sometimes of the apprentice's parent (P). After entering all the records in computer files came the critical task of splitting each record into two or three, with each name in turn at the head, so that all would appear in the alphabetical list. The licence records were relatively straightforward to add. From the Project's subscription files of some third-of-a-million names, those with a medical designation were extracted, condensed into one if the name of the medic appeared more than once, and added to the main sequence; the whole was then sorted alphabetically. Frequently the master's record could be related to university *alumni* (U), subscriptions (S), or other miscellaneous records (Z), and combined to make a standard summary (SSS) entry. The sequence was laser-printed and photo-copied to provide the first, limited, edition, largely consisting of the massive *Register*[5] with six kinds of entry arranged according to the following table A.

Table A: Column Arrangement of *Register*

Date	Symbol	Names	Job	Address	General
	(A)	Apprentice (Parent)	Master	Notes	Name of Master
	(M)	Master(period/premium)	Master	Master	Name of Apprentice
	(P)	Parent	Parent	Parent	Name of Apprentice
	BIL	Licensee	Licensee	Licensee	(Reference)
	SUB	Subscriber	Subscriber	Subscriber	Indicator
	SSS	Names, degree, fellow	Medic	Medic	Subscriptions (refs)

The SSS references are in order (B,C,D,O,M,L) - see next paragraph

The A, M, P entries should be taken as a whole to give the full Public Record Office record. When the licence entry lacks an address, the diocese given by the reference has been inserted. The SUBscriber entries stand out as having no entry in the date column, the date being clear from the indicator in the final column. The fuller, standard SSS entries contain other biographical details, (possibly several) jobs, addresses, subscriptions and references. The standard references are in the order indicated, starting with **B** to indicate books/articles written, specific college entries for Cambridge (and **O**xford after **DNB** entries), **M** for Munk entries (fellows or licentiates), and **L** for a library sale catalogue. Our young adolescent seemed sturdy and promising.

Because of restrictions on computer use, publication could not be delayed to explore other sources. However the interest aroused and the unsatisfied demand for further copies, combined with the opportunity to convert the first edition files for micro use, led to a decision to integrate new material with the old.[6] How much time and effort that was to involve was not then fully appreciated, as more and more sources have been used. We hope that the greatly increased content, enhanced accuracy and improved appearance will justify the decision. Mention may be made of the improved ordering, using standardised spelling of names in an unprinted computer field, of an enlarged introduction fuller than this paper, and of a greatly extended bibliography indicating the many more sources used. Our adolescent has grown into a maturing and attractive adult.

Subscription Material

It is clearly impossible even to mention all the work done since 1972 in the book subscription field, and the medical historian not familiar with it is advised to read some of the relevant PHIBB material.[7] Nonetheless, it is worth repeating that a normal entry in a list might include the subscriber's names, degrees and titles, his vocation and address, and occasionally personal notes. Lists vary considerably in completeness and size, with about three hundred names being typical (while others may exceed a thousand). The following list has been chosen partly because it is short, but chiefly because of its intrinsic, but hardly recognised, importance; it is unusual in naming students who attended the author's medical lectures in London. The MDs of four subscribers have been added and details of the others can be found in the *Register*.

Table B: Edward Strother   *EUODIA* 1718 [718STO]

The Subscribers Names, in the Order they Subscrib'd

Mr Edward Pearce, *Holsworth, Devon*
Mr William Norman, *Gilford, Surrey*
Mr J.Conningham, *Lugd.Bat. Penrith, Cumberland* [MD(R)1719]
Rufus Langley, *Newton-Abbot, Dev.*
James Briett, *Exeter, Devon*
Alexander Popham, *Exeter, Devon*
Edward Kenion, *Rochdale, Lancashire*
John Heathcote, *Lugd.Bat. Cut-Thorp, Derbyshire*
Daniel Flexney, *Lugd.Bat. Whitney, Oxon*
Cornelius Heathcote, *Cut-Thorp, Derbyshire*
John Challoner, *Morpeth, Northumberland*

Mr James Graham, *Lugd.Bat. Luckerby, Anandale* [MD(R)1718]
John Woodrow, *Lugd.Bat. Glasgow* [MD(R)1718]
Thomas Wilsford, *Cantab.Pontfract, Yorkshire* [MD 1728]
William Pennicott, *Sheer-Lane, London*
John Clarke, *Oxford, Oxon*
L. Holker, *Cantab. Gravesend, Kent*
John Rutherford, *Lugd.Bat. Edenborough*
—— Peck, *Drury-Lane, London*
William Musgrave, *Newcastle upon Tine*
Francis Dunn, *Alnwick, Northumberland*
George Story, *Newcastle upon Tine*
Richard Bishoppe, *Gravesend, Kent*
Willi Wymond, *Bodmin, Cornwall*
Benjamin Waide, *Hull, Yorkshire*
G. Locke, *Alnwick, Northumberland*

These Lectures were Finish'd in Seven or Eight Weeks.

Strother was born in Morpeth, Northumberland, and moved to Newcastle before settling in London. The close connection with Leyden (Lugd.Bat.) is significant, although it is not known whether Strother's MD, recorded on the title-page, was obtained there. Nor is any connection with Devon known, but the list shows clearly the significance of his lecturing to future graduates. For reference purposes this list has the indicator 718STO; the numbers refer to the date (1718); usually the letters are the first three of the author's name, but sometimes, as in this case, it is necessary to choose another appropriate final letter to make the indicator unique. Fuller details of this and other books can be obtained from the *Guide* and *Supplements*.[8] The original 1974 article was manually extracted from less than a hundred subscription lists, contrasting with over 1,100 lists giving nearly 400 thousand entries in the 1983 eighteenth-century subscription computer merge;[9] here mention may be made of the bias towards the early part of the century, with less than a quarter in the second half. A computer filter of the century merge gave ten thousand medical entries.

Sampling and Classification

To analyse fully all the material in the *Register* would have considerably delayed publication, so a 2% sample has been used. Computer filing throws together the (M) entries for different apprentices of the same master, perhaps as many as eight, but usually only a few, averaging 1.7. The records of many apprenticeships are not extant[10]; the sample shows that only 30% of functioning masters have their own apprenticeship recorded in the *Register*. One of the largest summary (SSS) entries is that for the influential Whig bibliophile, Richard Mead MD, who subscribed for some 200 books, but the largest in the sample is William Oliver of Bath with 25, and the average was 2.4 books per subscriber. Returns for parents not known to be medics (the correlation between parents' and sons' careers is worthy of separate study) and those licensed well before the eighteenth century are not included in the analysis, which indicates a total of over 35 thousand, a 50% increase over the first edition, with a distribution shown by table C and the diagram. Letters M,S,U,Z stand for master, subscribers, university, miscellaneous (next paragraph) entries, alone or in combination, as shown in the diagram.

Table C: Classification of Practising Medics
Figures based on 2% sample, adjusted to total 40

MS	SU	M only	S only	U only	Z	Total	M	S	U
2	4	9	5	4	16	40	11	11	8

The figures in the table have been simplified to give a total of 40 so that, approximately, multiplications by a thousand gives figures for the whole *Register*. The key result is that subscription entries are now as important as those from apprenticeships, and so justifies the emphasis given to them in this paper. University alumni are almost as significant, with half of them subscribers, twice as many as subscribing masters.

Miscellaneous Sources

Miscellaneous sources account for some 40% of the practitioners' entries in the *Register*, over four times as many as in the first edition. Not surprisingly this section is the fastest growing and should become more significant in the future. Starting with the specified B,D,M sources, some of the 78 bibliographical entries in the sample merely refer to copies of Edinburgh (and occasionally other university) theses; these contrast with an advertisement sheet by the Wakefield druggist, Thomas Lund (Table D). There must be many other similar ephemera which we would be delighted to hear about. The smaller (223 each) *DNB* and Munk entries are unlikely to grow as such, but further biographical sources could be more useful.

Emphasis has been put on combining national and local sources; the latter element is more difficult (if only because of the accessibility of material). Greater use has been made of institutional and local sources, such as parish registers, nonconformist and Church of England, and charity accounts. One advantage of using multiple sources is in the various descriptions of the tradesmen; one might give "draper" and another "apothecary", while one "Doctor" could be called "MD" in another. Recourse has been made to some regional (often county) pedigree collections, but these are usually too closely tied to visitation material and while indicating MDs, may ignore the less exalted surgeons and apothecaries, let alone paramedics. *Yorkshire Pedigrees*, by J.W. Walker[11] of Wakefield, is one of the more helpful.

Some medical readers may be surprised to see in the *Register* so many book tradesmen, although no doubt there should be more. Nowadays a bookseller is unlikely to print as well, and may sell only books. By contrast the eighteenth-century bookseller sold a great variety of other goods and provided many services. He often sold patent medicines and even dispensed drugs; in many ways he would act as the poor man's doctor and be the mainstay of self-medication, an important supplement to the traditional services. The tradesman often obtained much of his income from his medical work. For most today John Newbery is best known as a pioneer of children's books, but his biographer, Roscoe[12] suspects that he profited more from his medicines. His son, Francis junior, even withdrew from the book business to become a country gentleman, almost a millionaire, based on the profits of the Medical Warehouse by St Paul's and widespread dissemination of the patent medicines throughout the country. Alden's pioneer article[13] shows how widespread was the practice of provincial (and London) booksellers including patent medicines in their wares at the beginning of our period. More recently P.S. Brown[14] has given the results from Bath newspapers 1744-99, incidentally showing the considerable Newbery influence, and the value of any early local newspapers.

Desirable as it would have been, it has not been possible to include references to all the sources in each entry without extending the size and cost of the *Register*. Apart from the specific authorities given in SSS entries, some references can be inferred indirectly and it is hoped that the Medics Bibliography will enable a reader interested in a particular person to check the entry. In any case, the entry only summarises the information available in the Project's records; enquiries may be made of the authors, who will also be pleased to receive additions and corrections.

Places of Practice

The computer-produced topographical index gives the pages where there are references to a county or its chief towns and will be useful for a reader interested in a particular place. It cannot be used for statistical comparison because it does not indicate the number or nature of the occurrences on the page. The 2% sample shows that the leading English counties are: Lancashire, Devon, Kent, Essex, Leics, Lincs and West Riding, with Bristol the leading city. The more general analysis into Metropolitan, provincial, Scottish, Irish and Overseas practitioners, showing over twice as many provincial as metropolitan returns, may underestimate the real difference.

Table D: Wakefield Eighteenth Century Medics *(from PHIBB's Eighteenth Century Medics. 1988[6])*.

```
                                               A M              Subscriptions

b1650  1730 BARBER,Abraham      B PMed                  704HAR 710HAR 718PRI 720BEV 721SEN 730BED 730GEN
       1659 1726 WATKINSON,Benjamin  MD(O)
       1663 a1713 HATFIELD,Owen      Ap   Stanley
       1667 1733 MOORE,Thomas        MB(C) 'MD' Kirkgate
       1678 a1713 SCOTT,John         Ap
b1680  a1722 WADDINGTON,John     S Ap           (+4) 13 16 16 17 20 22
       1685 a1720 WILSON,Benjamin    Ap
       1687 a1713 LAWTON,Robert      Ap          A*
       1688 1775 WALKER,Thomas       S Ap         44 53 73
       1690 1752 HORNCASTLE,Richard  S   left for Huddersfield A*        733MAS
       1693 1767 WATKINSON,Edward    MD(U)  Minister (away)
b1695  a1718 CO(W)PE(R),John     S Ap          15 17 18
       1699 a1758 HOLME,Thomas       S           22 30 33 37 41 44        751BLE
       1699 1739 SLATER,Thomas       S Ap                                734SHO
b1700  a1720 BARGH,Mary          Ap Grocer       20
b1700  a1730 PERKINS,John        MD  Netherton
b1700  a1720 TILSON,John         Ap           18 20
b1700  1740 WALKER,William I     S             31                        734SHO
       1700 1779 COOKSON,John         MB(C) 'MD'                          734SHO 748WAR 778MAL
       1705 a1732 WILSON,Thomas       Ap          A 32
       1708 1768 HODGSON,Christopher  MD(C)
       1713 1773 STEER,Robert         S           47
       1722 1781 CHEETHAM,Robert      Ap S        A 55 60
H      1730 1805 AMORY,Robert         MB(C)         748RUT 748SAL 757OCK 759BUT 768HOU 782MOX 789LIN 802FRA

       1734 1791 ELLISON,John        S MD(X) Woolley  A 66              789LIN
       1738 1795 AMBLER,Richard      D grocer         69
b1740  1761 CLAPHAM,Thomas       Ap               61
       1742 1795 WALKER,William II   S Ap             82                 782MOX 788HAL 789LIN
b1745  1764 HOLDSWORTH,Thomas    MD(E)                                   764CRO
       1745 a1783 BOOTH,Richard       S Ap            A                  782MOX
H      1745 1820 RICHARDSON,James     MD(E) Dispensary Northgate            782MOX 789LIN 809BAW
       1747 a1791 COCKERILL,Theophilus S            A 77 91             '782MOX 789LIN
H      1753 a1826 DAWSON,William      MB(C) 'MD'MRCS JP Dispensary merchant 775CUT 776HUN 782MOX 789LIN 796JON 826ALE
H      1754 1814 TAYLOR,Edward        S Ap          75 83 89 91 93 96 02
b1755  a1775 LUND,Thomas         CD
       1755 a1783 KITSON,William      S            A                   782MOX
b1760  a1800 EARNSHAW,Richard    CD                83 96 00
b1760  a1826 HUERTLEY,Richard Henry MRCS left Wakefield 1784
b1760  a1811 LAWTON,William      CD Market Pl      A 83 88              811TIN
H b1760 1818 MITCHELL,William    S Ap Dispensary    81 05
       1762 a1812 STOTT,William       S
H      1766 1839 STATTER,Squire       S  Kirkgate       A               ?826ALE
       1768 a1822 RAMSBOTHAM,John MRCS after leaving   A
H      1769 1844 ALEXANDER,Disney  MD physician, author Dispensary Lupset Cottage,Kirkgate  802ATM
H b1770 a1839 HAIGH,     <Dame>  midwife Westgate
H      1772 1849 CROWTHER,Caleb      MD(E) Dispensary  Northgate,Kirkgate  805HOF
H      1772 a1822 THOMAS,Samuel       S                                814TIN
H b1775 a1837 HOLDSWORTH,William  Ap Dispensary
H      1775 1809 HOLDSWORTH,John      S  Kirkgate        A 05
H      1778 1855 WALKER,Benjamin    MRCS Westgate        A
H          a1853 WALKER,Ebenezer    MRCS Wood St, Albert Terrace          826ALE
b1780  a1802 FIELD,Robert        C    Westgate       02
b1780  a1801 KERSHAW,John        D    Silver St      01
H      1780 1825 MILNER,Richard       MRCS  Kirkgate

b1785  a1827 ELLIS,William Charles <Kt> MD MRCS  S  Asylum           826ALE
b1785  a1805 KERSHAW,Thomas      CD  Pig Market
b1785  a1822 POTTER,John         CD Market Pl,Westgate
H b1785 a1822 WALKER,William     S Ap (& STOTT,T)  Westgate  nd
H      1785 1832 REINHARDT,George B.  CD  Westgate      A 00            811TIN
H b1785 1828 STOTT,Thomas         S                                    826ALE
H      1786 a1871 THOMAS,William     MD(E) armyS Dispensary             826ALE
H          1809 BARBER,J.            C    Silver St
H b1790 1863 BENNETT,Joseph MRCS (& MILNER,R) Westgate A               826ALE 844LES
H b1790 a1853 MARSHALL,Samuel      S    Westgate
H b1795 a1841 TAYLOR,Edward II      S    Kirkgate
H      1797 1859 HORSFALL,John        S Dispensary Kirkgate,S Parade     826ALE
H b1800 1822 BIRKETT,John         Ap S D   Market Place
```

Wakefield has been chosen as an example, partly because the story summarised in table D complements that in Marland's recent book [15] and provides the background for her 1780-1870 account. H in the table indicates those mentioned by Marland[15] (who has kindly supplemented our first draft) and shows the overlap, as many of our practitioners lived on into the next century. The arrangement may be explained by the example of Theophilus Cockerill, not mentioned by Marland, born in 1747 and dying after 1791; he was a surgeon whose own apprenticeship and also two he took are recorded, and finally come two subscriptions.

The column headings A and M cover apprenticeship, and master having apprentices in the years (abbreviated by omitting the hundreds) stated. The additional Waddington apprenticeships are from a 1713 Exchequer case. Standard indicators show book subscriptions. Abraham Barber was a bookseller who also stocked patent medicines. The distribution is summarised in table E.

Table E: Distribution of Wakefield Eighteenth-Century Medics

Period	Physicians	Surgeon-Apothecaries	Qualified	Druggists	Total
Early	10	17	27	-	28
Later	6	21	27	9	37
Total above	16	38	54	9	65
Table total	18	48	66	11	79
Med.Register					
1780	*4*	*6*	*10*		

Cursory inspection of this table shows that the early nineteenth-century expansion described by Marland and others had begun much earlier. Considering the middle group, there are nine chemist/druggists compared with 27 qualified men, giving a ratio of 1:3, fitting Marland's varying from 1:3 in 1822 to equality half a century later. It will be noticed that four of the nine in the table occur only because of their apprentices. With small numbers it is more accurate to consider samples over a period than at a specific date, like the 1780 *Medical Register*.

For the whole century, the apprenticeships (not always at Wakefield) of 16 of the 48 surgeon-apothecaries are recorded, and 18 have apprentices of their own, underlining the importance of these records in the *Register*. These records are clearly usefully supplemented by subscriptions by 32; among the thirteen subscribing physicians is the leading, and long-living, Robert Amory (8 books). Not surprisingly, the one bookseller included was a frequent subscriber (7 books). The weight of subscription evidence would have been greater if the local book trade had developed earlier, and also if more later subscriptions had been analysed. It seems a little surprising that three medics bought the 1734 book of Thomas Short of Sheffield, but none bought the later ones. The seven copies of Moxon's *Most agreeable coompanion* and the five subscriptions to Linnecar's *Miscellaneous works* were due to the local influence of Wakefield authors. The final subscriptions were to two books by the local farrier John Tindall, and particularly (8 copies) to the 1826 *Lectures* by a Wakefield medic, Disney Alexander, printed and sold in Wakefield, an illustration of the need to consult post-1800 material to tell the complete eighteenth-century story.[16]

The records in the *Register*, largely from national sources not previously co-ordinated, give a coverage comparable with that obtained by detailed local research of particular towns in any of the four UK countr ies; further, for most of the century the information now made available is unique, since directories and census returns only appeared at the end.

Fuller details of many relevant subscription books mentioned can be found in Appendix IV of Medics with the titles and number of subscriptions of nearly a hundred lists by a variety (indicated) of medical authors, including a few in the early nineteenth century. It must not be assumed that all the subscribers to these books were medics - 718STO was an exception; also, of course, very many medics subscribed to other works detailed in the Project's *Guide*[8] Clearly the books to which medics subscribed give information about them. Even in this account of Wakefield medics, it has not been possible to analyse the significance of the subscription lists; a new approach had to be developed. By analysing the connections between the subscribers and their books, the Social Index gives numerical measures of different aspects or factors. Not surprisingly the most important is the temporal (clearly the bookseller Abraham Barber who died in 1730 could not have bought Thomas Short's 1767 book). The influence of topographical factors has already been indicated several times. Apart from medical and other scientific interests, the Index also measures cultural interests like music, religious and political views[17] When this work has been completed the medic will be seen in his full contemporary context.

Conclusions and Prospects

The vast amount of information presented in concise form in the *Register* will serve as an invaluable reference source, primarily for those interested in medical history. It shows both the essential use of computers and some of the problems involved. The preliminary sample analysis indicates some of the many aspects, including the size and geographical spread of the nascent profession, its nature and university connections, many apprenticeship practices, development during the century, literary and cultural interests shown by book subscriptions. Other users of the *Register* will include those with interests in the wider fields of the history of science and culture generally and more specifically of education, in urban history and local research, in prosopographical and genealogical studies, and other more particular themes like migration movements.

In his review of the first edition, Roy Porter expected it to stimulate "fine-textured surveys of the emergent medical profession", so it may be helpful to indicate a number of topics (many mentioned above) which could be developed from the present work and possibly help to improve its coverage. Several correspondents used the first edition for biographies of individuals or of particular families in which they were interested, aided by the additional material available at Newcastle. The treatment of Wakefield given briefly above could be paralleled by studies of many other regions or cities, which could be compared with Wakefield and also help to estimate the completeness of the *Register*. Taking the country as a whole, the geographical spread could be analysed to show gaps in the medical provision; arrangements in Wales as a whole would be interesting. The information in this *Register* could be worked up to make a much-needed biographical register of the significant Edinburgh medics. There are many problems which were not worth tackling in the small sample, but could provide worth-while results on a larger scale; as a start, it would be better to increase the 2% sample, perhaps first with a similar sample so that the new results could be compared with those above. Topics could include opticians and midwives, army surgeons, graduate surgeons, variations in parents' occupations and medics' schooling, books by or sale catalogues of medics. The significance of the preliminary analysis of changes during the century would be greatly strengthened by using the whole *Register* instead of the small sample. A full study of army surgeons, combining *Register* entries with Drew's army records, would yield important information on the growth of the profession. Without waiting for the full development of the Social Index, some readers might like to extend the work using subscriptions, such as those on individuals, comparing medical and other interests, or on readers of specific medical books.

Despite our pride in the achievements made, with due humility it is clear that with the co-operation of readers it should be possible to make a significant improvement. Many dates could be closed with knowledge of birth and death, and temporal extension may also give new addresses. Analysis of continental registers should reduce the number of unattributed MDs. Better coverage of Irish and particularly American sources would be a useful enhancement. More attention will be given to the various paramedics, especially those who helped with self-medication. It is hoped to remove the early bias of the subscriptions by more work on later lists, including some in the early part of the nineteenth century. Much stress has been laid above on further work on local sources to improve some of the entries given here. Similarly, the returns of many West Indian medics, usually from English sources, would be improved by a study of West Indian biographical material. More books and particularly articles, beyond those consulted and listed in the bibliography, should improve the existing entries and provide additional medics. Better referencing of individual entries should be seriously considered.

Readers' assistance is solicited and their comments on these and other points will be welcomed by the authors, to help the young adult to blossom, growing in experience and maturity.

Notes including Brief Bibliography and Relevant statistics extracted from P360

Figures in brackets refer to PHIBB reference numbers

1.   (B76) Book subscription lists *The Library* (5) **29**; p 3. A 1972 lecture, complementing B75 1979 (P196) *Book subscriptions - progress and plans*. A simple introduction, 1974

2.   (B66) *A preliminary guide to apothecaries in book subscription lists*, 322 names from 100 lists, 1974

3.   PRO Inland Revenue (medical) apprenticeships 50,000.

4.   Haggis Bishops' Licences. 4,285

5.   (P347) *Eighteenth century Medics* (1) contains 70,000 entries and nearly 25,000 practitioners

6.   (P360) *Eighteenth century Medics* (2) contains 80,000 improved entries and over 35,000 practitioners, a 50% increase. Appendices II and IV are the Selective Bibliography and Medical Subscription Lists, 1985

7.   (P356d) *Publications in Historical Bibliography*, giving other PHIBB items - available on request, 1987

8.   (B75) *Book subscription lists: a revised guide* (with 4 *Supplements*) - still available. After a comprehensive introduction come indicators and details of nearly 4,000 lists, 1975

9.   (P326) Eighteenth century subscription merge with 378,531 entries from 842 + 270 = 1,112 subscription lists for the two halves and the whole century - 9,387 medical entries, 1983

10.   Burnby, J.G.L. Apprenticeship records. *Trans Br Soc Hist Pharmacy* **i.** p4, 1977

11.   Walker, J.W. *Yorkshire Pedigrees* 3 vol (Harleian Society), 1942-4

12.   Roscoe, S. *John Newberg and his successors,* Wormley, 1973

13.   Alden, J. Pills and publishing ...1660-1725. *The Library* 5 **29,** p1,1952

14.   Brown, P.S. The Vendors of medicines advertised in eighteenth century Bath newspapers. *Medical History* **19,** p3, 1975

15.   Marland, H. *Medicine and society in Wakefield and Huddersfield 1780-1870,* Cambridge, 1987

16.   Reference to books mentioned in the text, with the PHIBB reference code in brackets.
Moxon, J. *Most agreeable coompanion* (ii) Leeds 1782. (782MOX)
Linnecar, R. *Miscellaneous works* . . . Leeds 1789. (789LIN)
Tindall, J. *Observations of the breeding . . . of neat cattle* Leeds 1811. (811 TIN)
Tindall, J. *...'s Yorkshire farriery,* Huddersfield 1814. (814 TIN)
Alexander, D. *Lecture on phrenology,* London, Edinburgh and Wakefield 1826. (826 ALE)

17.   *Social index calculations* 1984

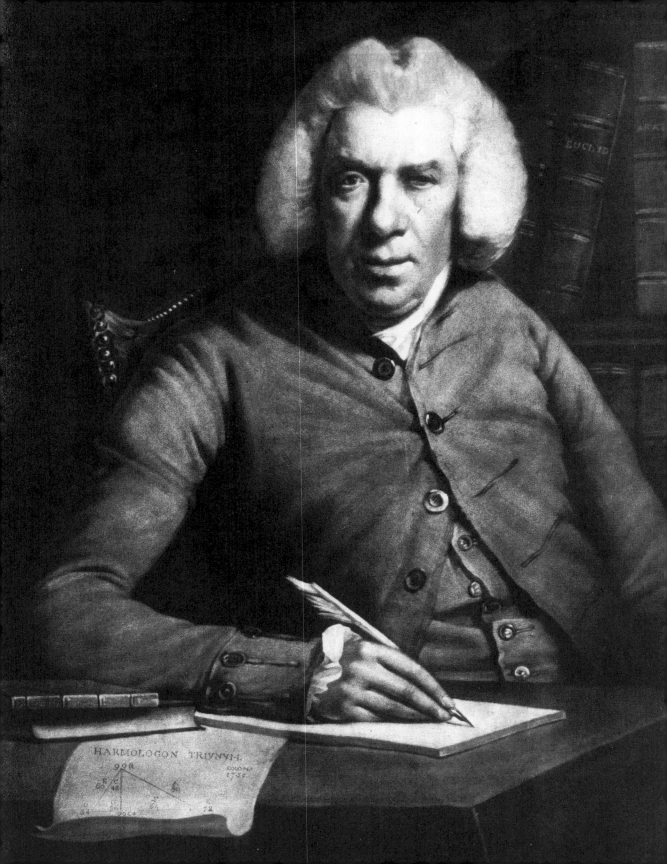

HARMOLOGON TRIVNVM.

WEAVING A WEB AROUND DR HENRY HARINGTON

Sholem Glaser

Henry Harington was born at Kelston, near Bath, in September 1727. His ancestors include one John Harington, treasurer to Henry VIII's camps and buildings, who acquired the family estates at Kelston, and who had a son, another John, famous for his wit and his water closet. Henry Harington's father was the last of the family to live at Kelston, disposing of the estate in 1759 to Mr Hawkins, later Sir Caesar Hawkins, surgeon to Georges II and III.

Henry Harington received his early education at home from the Rev Dr Fothergill. He then went to live with his uncle, the Rev William Harington, vicar of Kingston in Wiltshire, who arranged for his entry to Queen's College Oxford in 1745. While living with his uncle Henry began composing music, including a duet called *Damon and Clora*. He also wrote various odes, among them the *Witch of Wokey* which is mentioned in all biographical notes and was apparently quoted in many contemporary anthologies.

In addition he wrote prologues and epilogues for two rival theatres in Bath, one located in North Parade under the Lower Assembly Rooms and the other, the New Theatre, situated in Kingsmead Street where it functioned between 1723 and 1751.

Harington graduated in 1749 but decided not to seek holy orders. He turned his attention to the study of physic, encouraged by an uncle in Bath, Dr Edward Harington (1696-1757), who was physician to the Bath Hospital (ie Royal Mineral Water Hospital) 1740-1750. J.R. Magrath, the author of the standard history of the Queen's College, mentions that Harington was one of several College members who, in 1748, broke the rule which required them to dine in hall. What sounds a trivial enough episode developed into a pamphlet war, and some of the College members, but not Harington, withdrew from Queen's. He remained at Oxford to take his MA in 1752 and proceeded to Bachelor and Doctor of Medicine in 1762. He appears to have been something of a polymath - a good classical scholar, good at literature, interested in mechanical inventions, mathematics and astronomy. But his main interest was music. It will no doubt be noticed that the only subject not listed in his various activities and interests is medicine. While at Oxford he joined an amateur musical society to which were admitted only those who were able to play and sing at sight.

He left Oxford for Wells in 1753 where he practised medicine. It is interesting to note that he started to practise in 1753 but only received his medical degree in 1762. He was the only doctor there and apparently felt cut off from colleagues, so he moved to Bath in 1771 to follow his uncle. None of the writers of his obituaries or biographies appear to have been very interested in his medical career. There may be sources of information as yet

40. (left). Dr Henry Harington. An engraving by Charles Turner after a portrait by Thomas Beach. 1799. *(By courtesy of Clive Quinnell)*

undiscovered. He was certainly physician to the Mineral Water Hospital, 1780-1799. It is said that his house was open on certain days to the poor for advice, and he was willing to send advice by post to those who sought it.

The Duke and Duchess of York were frequent visitors to Bath. The Duke was a member of the Harmonic Society (of which more later) and Dr Harington was appointed as their physician. He was also physician and close friend of the Piozzi family and looked after them for many years. He married "the amicable and accomplished Miss Musgrave of Oxford". They had four children, three sons and one daughter. His daughter Susan Isabella married Archdeacon Josiah Thomas and lived in Bath. Archdeacon Thomas appears to have written a memoir of Dr Harington during his life-time, but the Bath Reference Library has no reference to this in its index and was unable to trace it; it is doubtful whether it would have contained anything of medical interest.

Harington served the town as Alderman and Magistrate and was appointed Mayor on 1st November 1793. The Minutes of his year of office deal largely with regulations of hackney coaches, chairs and chairmen, leases of property, payments to architects and builders eg, Mr Palmer consulted about completing the elevation of the Pump Room. Also we find regulations for navigation from Newbury to Bath on the Kennet and Avon Canal, and alterations to the gaol "for the better securing of prisoners". The Mayor had usually been given a stipend of £105. In September it was decided to increase it to £420 out of which the Mayor had to pay for the two usual entertainments and every other usual expense attending his Mayoralty. There is only one medical minute, namely that in September 1794 Joseph Phillott, Surgeon, was elected surgeon to Bellott's Hospital or Almshouse in place of Henry Wright deceased.

Henry Harington was concerned with the erection of Northumberland Buildings where he lived and where he died in 1816 aged 89. Murch recalls that sixty years before writing his book he often met people who remembered Dr Harington - his general good manners, his agreeable conversation, and his rich store of anecdotes. Others remembered him not long before his death sitting at Bull's Library in his full bottomed wig, with his three-cornered hat, completely blind, chatting sociably and full of animation. He was buried in Kelston but his monument is in the Abbey. His eldest son Edward was also Mayor of Bath and was knighted by George III. His second son Henry became a prebendary of Wells and then moved on to various posts in Norwich. Dr Henry Harington was best known in his lifetime and best remembered after his death for his musical activities, though clearly his appointments to the Mineral Water Hospital and as a physician to the Duke of York suggest that his medical reputation must also have been good. He is said to have devoted all his leisure to music and literature.

During the period with which we are dealing Bath had an active musical circle. The names that spring to mind are the Linleys and the Herschels (William and his sister Caroline) but there were many others not so well remembered now. Among these Rauzzini must be specially noted. Dr Harington and his friends revived a decaying catch club and from it formed the Bath Harmonic Society. In 1784 he was appointed physician to the Harmonic Society, which thrived and became very popular though select. "None but gentlemen of known character were proposed and balloted for". Members included George IV and the Duke of York. The Society met every Friday during the winter and spring - there was a cold supper and much conviviality after. Between 1780 and 1800 Dr Harington published four collections of musical compositions especially glees, elegies and canons.

The word glee was derived from the old English "gleo" meaning music, and is not generally associated with mirth. A glee is a choral composition for unaccompanied male voices. The high period for glees was 1750 to 1830 and it is a purely English form. Glee clubs played a notable part in musical life during this period.

Harington gained great fame for his "Eloi" or "The Last Words of our Saviour" which was sung in Bath Abbey Church on Good Friday for many years, and which is represented on his monument. Apart from this he composed very little sacred music but one of his hymn tunes (Retirement) is still in use today in *Hymns and Psalms* 573 "When all thy mercies, O my God" and in *Songs of Praise* 613 "O sweeter than the marriage-feast".

In a small book by Harold Jeboult on *Somerset Composers, Musicians and Music*, a short account is given of Harington's musical activities. One not mentioned in other works is his association with the controversy surrounding the history of the National Anthem. He advocated the claim of Henry Carey (1692-1743) as its composer, a claim much favoured in America. Apparently Henry Carey himself did not claim to have written *God Save the King* and it was never included in his publications. It was his son who claimed that his father had written it in 1745 or 1746, but he had forgotten that his father had died in 1743.

Before ending this short biography here are a few quotations to give some idea of Dr Harington's literary efforts and humour. The best known is the amusing epigram usually described as "An impromptu by Dr Harington when walking in the Abbey at Bath".

> These ancient walls, with many a mouldring bust
> But show how well Bath Waters lay the dust.

He was also the author of the lines on Beau Nash's memorial in the abbey. Sometimes his humour was tinged with irony, or can it even be called cynicism, as shown in this short verse:

> War begets poverty, poverty peace,
> Peace makes riches flow, fate ne'er does cease.
> Riches produce pride, and pride is war's ground,
> War begets poverty, the world goes round.

He also published a Geometrical Demonstration of the Indivisibility of the Trinity under the title of *Symbolon Trisagion*. This is probably the reason for the triangle in his monument, which is one of the most beautiful in Bath Abbey. He also wrote the Stammering Glee which describes a man in haste enquiring for a midwife and being delayed by two stammerers each giving him different directions.

He himself was the subject of a eulogy in verse:

On H. Harington of Bath MD

Last of that old and honour'd race, whose name
Stands high upon their country's roll of fame,
The good shall mourn thee, Harington; but most,
They, who thy love for lettered art may boast,
Who stoop to drink from clear Castalie's well,
Or listen to the full and solemn swell
Of Music's sweetest mood!
          One daughter's tear
That wets the grave of Him, whom ALL revere,
Shall shew, though aged, thou didst not survive
Those best and holiest sympathies, that live
In silent duty's heart!
          Heav'n seem'd to spare,
Thy term of days, though mark'd, alas! with care,
That children of a later age might trace
The gentler virtues of thy ancient race.
Oppress'd by almost ninety years, and blind;
BEHOLD THE CHRISTIAN! STRICKEN, YET RESIGNED!
Sleep the long night of death, beneath this stone!
The strain that wakes thee next, may seem thy own!

An obituary in a London paper in January 1816 shows that he was well known as a musician:

"Dr Harington of Bath (whose death we announced last week) was descended from an ancient and honourable family, who long possessed considerable influence and property in the neighbourhood; he had become identified in a manner with the town, and appeared a venerable yet graceful antiquity amidst its modern refinements. The mildness and suavity of his address and deportment, his gentlemanly manners, his talents, his acquirements and a large fund of anecdotal recollections, rendered him a companion at once delightful and instructive. His name in the musical world stands deservedly high as a composer; and without being a performer on any instrument he thoroughly understood the science of music. His productions, whether humorous or grave, whether light or sacred, from the festive catch to the sublime Eloi, alike display the refined taste of a connoisseur, and the powerful conception of a master. Perfectly familiar with classical literature, Dr Harington was equalled by few as a general scholar and his Latin compositions were distinguished by their purity and elegance. Some exquisite specimens in his native tongue prove that he possessed in no mean degree the requisites of a poet. His passage through life exemplified the mild influence of the religion he professed; and his death, without pain and without a struggle, gave to his surviving friends a true spectacle of the Christian Euthanasia."

Finally, here is an unusual laudatory appreciation:

> His philanthropy and charity were unbounded: and his feelings towards the brute creation extended to so great a degree, that he left in his will one guinea per annum for an annual sermon to enforce the practice of humanity to brute animals.

Bath's social pre-eminence in the latter half of the 18th century was matched by a large active medical community. Most notable was Caleb Hillier Parry who was closely associated with Jenner at Berkeley and who with others in the area formed the Medico-Convivial Club which met at the 'Fleece.' One of the most important topics discussed was the association of angina pectoris with disease of the coronary arteries. There is the well documented relationship between John Hunter and Edward Jenner. We know that Jenner and Parry were close friends. In fact Jenner dedicated *An Enquiry into the Causes and Effects of the Variolae Vaccinae* to C.H. Parry at Bath. Equally well known is that John Hunter suffered from angina and on more than one occasion came to Bath to convalesce, and that Jenner came over from Berkeley to visit him. The unsolved question is who actually looked after Hunter in Bath.

It has been accepted usually that Hunter visited Bath twice - in 1777 and 1785. It is certain, however, that he came here four times at least. David Hume the philosopher wrote from Bath on 10th June 1776 that he had consulted John Hunter "coming accidently to town". Hume died later that year from cancer, so there can be no mistake about the year. Hunter had suffered from angina for three years and this seems to have been his first bad attack and his first stay in Bath. His second visit in 1777 after another attack is well recorded by his letters to Jenner from Bath. In August 1777 a letter to Jenner announces his intention to set out for Bath. He returned to London via Southampton in "less than three months" so presumably he was in Bath for quite a long time, probably until November. His third visit was two years later in 1779. A letter written in November 1779 from London states "Mrs Hunter and I were at Bath the other day, and came home by way of Gloucester". As in the case of the first visit no details have been found as to how long they stayed in Bath. And finally his fourth visit was in 1785 when there is a letter of this date from Anne Hunter in Bath to Jenner. On this occasion they stayed three to four weeks, and it is this visit that is commemorated by a plaque at No 12 South Parade.

So who looked after Hunter? For a moment it looked as if the problem had been solved when Le Fanu published his *Biobibliography of Edward Jenner*. In it he states:- "He (Hunter) went to Bath where Parry looked after him from August to November 1777". However this was pure conjecture for which he had no evidence. In fact Parry was still a medical student in Edinburgh when Hunter first came to Bath. This error was repeated some years later when the *British Journal of Surgery* reprinted Hunter's letters to Jenner. Following correspondence with the editor the mistake was corrected when the letters were published as a book. There is some evidence that Parry looked after John Hunter on his fourth visit in 1785 when he stayed at No 12 South Parade. Who looked after Hunter on his visits in 1776, 1777 and 1779?

About thirty years ago two prints came up for sale in a local Bath auction room. One was of the Reynolds portrait of John Hunter and the other was of Dr Henry Harington from the portrait by Thomas Beach. They were bought and hung on my wall almost unnoticed until recently. (The Harington print has been given to the Royal National Hospital for Rheumatic Diseases as they had no portrait of him).

In 1983 the Holburne of Menstrie museum put on an exhibition based on the visit of Haydn to Bath in 1794. It was his second visit to England. Haydn came to Bath on 2nd August for a few days and stayed with his friend Venanzio Rauzzini in Perrymead. Rauzzini had been a famous composer and castrato singer. Mozart who heard Rauzzini in Italy was so impressed that he wrote the motet *Exultate, Jubilate* for him. He left Italy for London and, after a successful career there, retired from the stage and settled in Bath, where he taught singing and organised subscription concerts in the New Assembly Rooms. While in Bath Haydn met Dr Henry Harington and apparently was impressed by his verses and compositions. Harington wrote a verse of praise for Haydn which the latter set to music (a combination of soprano solo, four part chorus - two sopranos, tenor and bass - and pianoforte) which was published in Leipzig in 1806 under the title *Dr Harington's Compliment*.

As already stated one of the few things known about Dr Harington's medical activities is that he was physician and friend to the Piozzi family. Mrs Thrale, the friend of Dr Samuel Johnson, came to Bath in 1781 after the death of Mr Thrale and settled at 8 Gay Street. In 1784 she married Mr Piozzi at St James Church. They lived in various homes in Bath - Alfred Street, Bennett Street, 43 Pulteney Street and others.

It was while looking at Henry Harington's portrait in the Holborne Museum exhibition that one was reminded that Anne Hunter - John's wife - also had some connection with Haydn, whom she had met in London. She had written most of the libretti for a dozen canzonettas that Haydn had composed while in London. These were performed in Bath in November 1794 having been harmonised by Rauzzini. She also wrote a libretto for *The Creation* but it was not accepted, another being preferred. And when Haydn left London she presented him with a farewell poem which he set to music.

Anne Hunter's social evenings were always crowded with well known people, and one of her friends and guests was Mrs Thrale. After one such evening Mrs Thrale wrote in her notebook "the heart of a frog will not cease to beat, says John Hunter, for four hours after it has been torn from the body of the animal".

Thus there are some coincidences. Firstly there is the appearance in the auction rooms of the two prints, Hunter and Harington; secondly two people Anne Hunter and Harington, both meeting Haydn, both presenting him with complimentary verses which he set to music; and finally, both Anne Hunter and Henry Harington being friendly with Mrs Thrale (Piozzi). Could Dr Harington have looked after Hunter? At the period of Hunter's first visits he was a leading if not *the* leading physician in Bath. But there is no cast iron evidence. Sadly the tantalising temptation to draw some conclusion from these tenuous coincidences has led nowhere. We remain tangled in the strands of the web around Dr Harington.

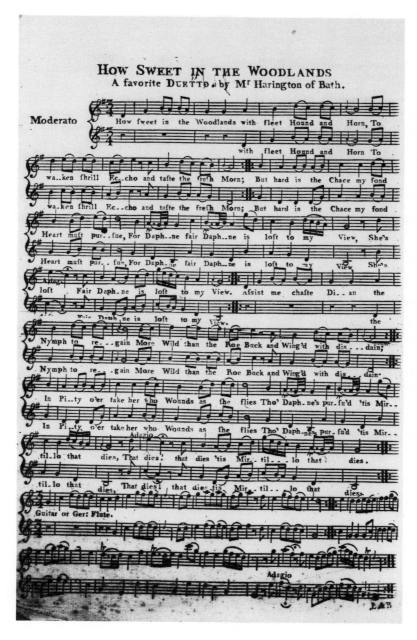

41. Musical score by Dr Harington. *(By courtesy of Clive Quinnell)*

BIBLIOGRAPHY

1.   Bath Municipal Archives

2.   *Dictionary of National Biography*, **24,** p 385

3.   Falconer, R.W. *History of the Royal Mineral Water Hospital*, Bath, 1888

4.   Grimble, I. *The Harington Family*, London, 1957

5.   Harington, H. Bath Anecdotes and Characters, London, 1782

6.   ibid, *Songs, Duets and other Compositions*. Collected by his daughter Susan Isabella Thomas, 1800

7.   *Haydn in Bath*, Holburne of Menstrie Museum, 1982

8.   Jeboult, H.A. *Somerset Composers, Musicians and Music*, Somerset Folk Series no 10, 1923

9.   LeFanu, W.R. A *Bio-Bibliography of Edward Jenner*, London, 1951

10.   Lowndes, W. *They Came to Bath*, Bristol, 1982

11.   ibid, *The Theatre Royal at Bath*, Bristol, 1982

12.   Murch, J. *Biographical Sketches of Bath Celebrities*, London, 1893,,

13.   Paget, S, *John Hunter*, London, 1897

14.   Philo-Musicus. Dr Harington, Biographical Sketch, *Bath and Bristol Magazine*, **3,** p 341, 1834

15.   Poynton, F.J. Kelston, a Village in Somerset, *St Barts Hosp Journal*, Jan 1933

16.   Quist, G. *John Hunter*, London, 1981

17.   Roberson, C. *Bath, An Architectural Guide*, London, 1975

18.   Sundry cuttings and letter. Bath Reference Library

MILTON'S DUBLIN EDITOR: EDWARD HILL, MD

J B Lyons

Edward Hill is an established minor figure in the annals of Irish medical history, King's professor of medicine in Dublin University and several times president of the College of Physicians. Most accounts of Hill dwell on his aspiration to provide a new and adequate botanical garden and the feud with Dr Robert Perceval who opposed him and merely mention his unpublished edition of *Paradise Lost*. This perspective is correct from a vocational viewpoint but I shall present his professional career briefly, taking his literary interests as the focus of my attention.

The eldest of Thomas and Mrs Hill's seven children, Edward Hill was born on 14 May 1741 near Ballyporeen, a County Tipperary village now rejoicing as President Reagan's ancestral place. The lad was tutored by a local clergyman until his father's death, when the family moved close to Cashel where he attended a classical school daily until ready to go as boarder to the Diocesan School of Clonmel.[1]

He entered Trinity College, Dublin in 1760, was elected Scholar in 1763 and graduated BA in 1765. His intellectual brilliance was crowned by exceptional calligraphy; the task of writing out a testimonium for the Duke of Bedford was deputed to him by the Board, his reward five guineas. Instead of seeking a fellowship, a distinction thought to be well within his powers, he turned to medicine. He took the MB degree in 1771, proceeded MD in 1773 and was elected Fellow of the College of Physicians two years later.

Little is known of his medical practice but he is said to have been particularly interested in sick children. Honours came to him swiftly. Before long Hill was lecturer in botany (1773), regius professor of physic (1781) which chair he retained for 49 years, and physician to Mercer's Hospital. Directly and indirectly he was involved with botany, the importance of which in medical treatment at that time cannot be over-rated. Just then, for instance, a Birmingham practitioner, Dr William Withering, having expertly selected foxglove as the active ingredient of a folk-cure, was about to introduce digitalis, a remedy still in daily use.

Hill was outraged to find that the physic garden available for him was a strip of rat-infested ground shadowed by the over-hanging branches of lofty elms and used as a dumping ground by the adjoining anatomy school, despite the supervision of an elderly gardener. He decided not to replace the old man when he died and approached the authorities for permission to use a vacant plot of ground at Townsend Street.

A *hortus sanitatis* was a traditional and, as Hill saw it, a necessary amenity for an eighteenth century medical school; others, and particularly those who had experienced teaching methods in Edinburgh and elsewhere abroad, believed that the provision of facilities for clinical teaching was a priority. The School of Physic Act of 1785 elevated Hill's botany lectureship to a chair but funds were set aside for clinical lectures and nothing for the garden.

Arrangements were made to reserve a ward for teaching in Mercer's Hospital. Later a house was rented in Clarendon Street but proved too costly and besides Dr Perceval, whom Hill described as "a self-sufficient, vindictive gentleman, singularly obstinate in his own opinion", wished to establish an institution resembling the Edinburgh Royal Infirmary.[2]

The University and the College of Physicians eventually agreed to co-operate in order to provide a physic garden. The physicians offered an annual sum of £100 from Sir Patrick Dun's estate. The legality of the use of Dun's monies was disputed. Legal opinions were sought, subcommittees formed and the agreement made in 1793 was reversed in 1798 by the chairman's casting vote. Meanwhile, confident of success and with the provost's approval, Hill had leased a six-acre field at Harold's Cross, prepared to pay half the rent until such time as the ground was required. When the College of Physicians withdrew its support, he decided to use his entire salary to fund the project but, in 1800, through the machinations of Perceval, the second School of Physic Act decreed that no person could hold two chairs and he was obliged to give up the chair of botany.

Finally, Hill went to law with the provost and fellows to recover his money. The case was tried at the King's Bench in March 1803 and Hill was awarded £618. Subsequently he published *An Address to the Students of Physic* (1803), an apologia containing a promise couched in a Miltonic metaphor - "Nor will I call from off the oblivious pool those Demons that have disturbed our primeval peace: those Spirits of malignant Passions, of Envy, Pride, Hypocrisy and mean Revenge".[3]

An unrepentant humanist at a time when medical writers were using the vernacular increasingly, Edward Hill's ears were closed to pleas that in the medical faculty, examinations should be conducted in English. So long as it was in his power to influence matters, he intended to resist this change. His preference for Latin as the conventional academic tongue reflects literary interests that led him to amass a splendid collection of books and to seek control of the university printing house.

T.P.C. Kirkpatrick's inference in his *History of the Medical School* that Hill needed increased space for his botany lectures is probably incorrect. However crowded the old Anatomy House may have been, it is unlikely that students would have been given the run of an area containing valuable machinery and types. And besides, Hill's comments indicate familiarity with printers' procedures. He complains, for instance, of an editor's "Being unacquainted with the operations and rules of printing" and refers to Baskerville's "hot-pressed pages".

Hill was given the use of the Printing House by the Board for five years in 1774. The period was extended and during the years of his occupancy he was joined by Joseph Hill (the relationship, if any, is unknown) who in 1779 printed Anthony Vieyra's *Animadversiones Philologicae*. This, as Vincent Kinane was pointed out, was the first of a series of scholarly works printed by Joseph Hill. Books on mathematics and science dominate but the list includes the first book from the press to use Hebrew type (Buxtorf's *Grammar,* 1782) and the first work in Italian to be printed in Ireland (Boiardo's *Orlando Inamorato,* 1784), the production of which was supervised by Dr Hill who bore the cost.

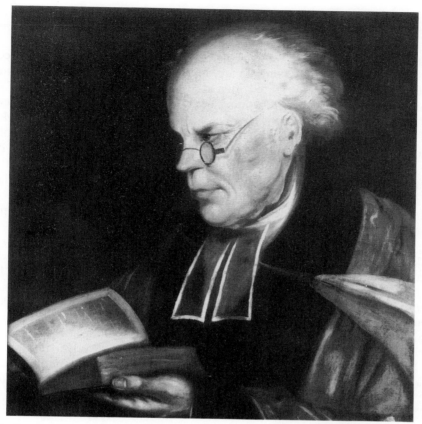

42. Portrait of Dr Hill. *(By courtesy of the Royal College of Physicians of Ireland)*

But by printing political tracts of a seditious nature, Joseph Hill put the Board in an embarrassing position. A meeting was arranged between the Chief Secretary, Thomas Orde, and Provost Hely Hutchinson, who was asked to account for the printer's activities. Writing to the provost on 27 August 1784, Orde expressed concern regarding "dangerous machinations in very dangerous quarters" and asked for Dr Hill's address. On the same day, "Dr Hill having ... at ye Board resigned the use of the Printing House & delivered up the key, the head porter was order'd to take possession of the Printing House".[4]

Nothing further is heard of the matter. Unlike a colleague, Whitley Stokes, who was deprived of a tutorship for favouring the United Irishmen, Edward Hill appears to have suffered no reprimand. One is inclined to see him as the printer's innocent associate but his Address inveighs against the Act of Union and an Assembly "who were then preparing to close their political existence by the barter of the Rights, the Property, and the Peace of their Country".

Hill's library, which he sold by auction in 1816, contained more than 1800 volumes. These included eighteen incunabula and 101 books printed in the first half of the sixteenth century. The wide range covered the Greek and Latin classics, Greek testaments, Hebrew bibles, French and Italian literature.[5]

From his youth, John Milton's writings had, as Hill put it, "obtained a preference" in his mind. "When chearful and devoid of care, I have resorted to them for amusement and instruction, and they have contributed often to console me in the hour of sorrow". Having read many editions of the poetical works closely, he was increasingly concerned by the number of ill-conceived alterations he noticed, particularly in *Paradise Lost*. He finally decided to republish the second edition of Paradise Lost printed in 1674 and embodying corrections made by Milton; to this end he collated it with several of the later editions.

He was twenty-eight when he embarked on his vocational undertaking which planned to include an index to the great poem. He finished it forty-four years later in 1813. The dull task of transcribing in his fine meticulous hand a fair copy of the index was completed on Thursday 29 July 1824.

The undated prospectus of A New and Correct Edition of Milton's *Paradise Lost* offered for 20s a work in two octavo volumes "handsomely printed on superfine paper" which was to be sent to press by Messrs Bentham and Hardy of Cecilia Street, booksellers, when a sufficient number of subscribers had been obtained. But for one reason or other it was never published and the manuscript was donated to Trinity College by his daughter, Mrs Curtis of Portlaw, County Waterford, in 1874. It has attracted little attention from literary scholars. Robert Bell, a former Trinity College alumnus and arts graduate who may have seen it in Hill's lifetime, referred to it in 1839 as "the most remarkable instance of devotion to the memory of a poet, to be found, perhaps, in the annals of literature", and

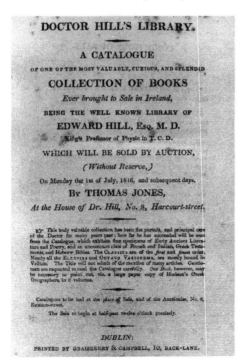

43. Catalogue for the auction sale of Dr Hill's library, 1816.. *(By courtesy of Trinity College, Dublin)*

called the Prolegomena "a masterpiece of critical disquisition".[6]   It is a remarkable exercise in polemics reminiscent in this respect of Dr James Henry's commentary on Virgil's *Aeneid*. James Henry read classics and medicine at Trinity College between 1817 and 1824 and may have been influenced by Hill.[7]

Hill's beautifully-written manuscript[8] comprises five copybooks containing a Prolegomena, a massive word-index to *Paradise Lost,* discussions on French translation and criticism, accounts of the engraved portraits of Milton and of plates used in the several editions. Tables of previous editors' errata are provided and an anthology of "the Censures and erroneous judgements, which Writers have pronounced on Milton". The fifth book contains Hill's notes on *Paradise Lost.* The alterations to be embodied in the new edition are written into his own interleaved copy of the 1674 edition.

He recalls in the Prolegomena how he became determined "to restore to the World the genuine Text of our unrival'd Poet, cleansed and purified from every adventitious foulness ...". With this intent he had read all the existing editions and could claim "a knowledge of their peculiarities, more minute and critical, than any Editor has ever hitherto applied any pains to obtain". He indulges no hypothesis, removes nothing and spares no labour in the endeavour to provide a standard for future editions.

He did not hope to attain fame, his sole purpose "to preserve the Text intire; and to absterge such blemishes as, from inadvertance or intention, have been infixed upon it". Printers and editors are castigated for errors and omissions which blemish the editions of *Paradise Lost* published since Milton's death. The printers facilitated "the mercenary usage of illiterate Booksellers"; the editors busied themselves in "splenetic Criticism" and in "the coacervation of futile, verbose Commentary". The third edition was hurried from the press in 1678 abounding in errors and Hill condemns the "atrocious injuries its Editor has committed, even to the enormity of leaving out an entire line, the 659th of the XIth Book".

The folio editions (1688, 1692, 1695) incorporating the errors of the third edition down to the missing line made Hill very angry. The seventh edition (1705) also is judged to be inferior but by some lucky casualty, the excluded line is reinstated. The eleventh edition is a worthless little book that should be thrown into a corner and Hill complains that "the muddy Torrent of abuses and corruptions become still more turbid as it flows on, each successive Edition being polluted by an increase of new mistakes ...".

Editors selected for particular disapprobation include Elijah Fenton, whose spelling and punctuation upset Hill, the Bishop of Bristol, Dr Thomas Newton, dismissed for superficiality, and Richard Bentley whose disrespect for Milton infuriated Hill, to whom *Paradise Lost* was "an emanation from nothing less than an immortal mind". Bentley believed that the proof-sheets of the first and second editions were never read to Milton "who, unless he was as deaf as blind, could not possibly let pass such gross and palpable Faults", and, though himself a septuagenarian, referred pityingly to "poor Milton in that Condition, with Three-score Years Weight upon his Shoulders, might be reckoned more than half Dead".

The Baskerville editions were praised for typographical beauty but Hill noted that John Baskerville, "the boast of his country - and its shame" was obliged to sell his type, implements and the secrets of his art abroad.

Then he expounded on the duties of the ideal editor:

> A judicious and conscientious Editor will treat his Author, as the skilful Artist, who, to repair a Picture, the Work of some great Master, Rafaelo or Corregio, with light and expert touches of his pencil, fills up and hides its accidental flaws and fissures, but will not superinduce new tints nor shades, to impair the perfections of the inimitable Tablet. Such an Editor will even spare some blemishes, which the Author, intent on more exalted contemplations, may have overpassed: and allows them to remain, as Spots may appear upon the disk of the Sun.

When preparing his own edition, Hill took the second edition for model - a book "worthy not of Cedar only, but to be inshrined in the rich-jewelled Coffer of Darius" - consulting the first edition "for the rectification of some few mistakes, which have been accidentally overlooked in the printing of the Second".

Even the pointing did not escape Hill's attention- "Nothing can more injuriously affect the sense of an Author's expressions than the wrong position of their points. Confusio punctis confunduntur omnia".

Towards the end of his abusive commentary he found praise for editions published in Dublin and based on the first and second editions - John Hawkey's edition (1747) "issued in much purity from the Press of the University of Dublin" and another from T. Ewing - but may have thought this passage smacked of chauvinism and deleted it.

He wondered why the earliest editions were so little used:

> The homely coarseness of their garb, devoid of every typographic decoration; (and which was soon outshone by the more imposing dream of specious Folios, or of other forms more trim from the printer's art, that usurped their juster rights,) may have principally caused this neglect; their mean appearance exciting but a feeble interest, and excellence being deemed commensurate with ornament.

The Index was completed after "drudging labor" in 1813. Robert Bell described it as "a marvellous exercise of human ingenuity - a task which ordinary powers could not have effected, and from which even great powers, associated with less energy, would have recoiled". Every word of the twelve books of Paradise Lost is incorporated and, where appropriate, subdivisions were used, eg read - participle; read - preterite; read - imperative; to read - infinitive.

Hill believed it would serve "as an absolute preservative of its Text, which, so long as this Index, constructed on the genuine Edition, shall continue in existence, can never more sustain abuse or corruption, without it being immediately and infallibly detected". With its aid he was enabled to call "the several tribes of Words" from "their distinct recesses throughout the volume", examine the orthography and when necessary impose corrections.

Variations could generally be explained by Milton's use of different amanuenses and Hill was not willing to accept the "methodical design" suspected by other editors. This is "chimerical" and he is prepared to impose uniformity.

> Yet there are some cases that must be excepted, to which even this becoming Uniformity cannot extend. The participle *been,* for instance, when it is to be pronounced quicker, is always bin: And the pronoun possessive *their,* which is the Saxon hir with a t prefixed, is therefore universally written thir by Milton, except in a few instances, where, the Verse requiring a more lengthened and emphatical pronounciation, it is *their,* in the commonly-received form. These distinctions seem to have been too evidently marked by the Author to admit any alteration.

Personal pronouns, he, me, she, we, ye, are written hee, mee, shee, wee, yee, when strong emphasis is required. Bell claims that Hill was the first to draw attention to Milton's use of orthographic variations to achieve variations of rhythm.

Was he the first to embark on a Miltonic word-index? Possibly, but others shared the intention and the Rev Henry Todd's edition of the Poetical Works (1809) contains an index which in addition to the general text covers Greek, Latin and Italian words.[9]

Hill approved of the German and Italian translations but said the French translations were "nothing better than the attempts of presumptuous ignorance to do what far excelled the powers of that meagre idiom to accomplish ..." He shows, with an almost audible snort, that the Abbé Delille has introduced references to Isaac Newton whose discoveries were not published until after Milton's death and charges him, in view of his substitution of thyme for fennel, with ignorance of what Pliny says "of the gratefulness of the smell of Fenel to Serpents" and of finding a new employment for Eve: " - With her belles mains the jeune beauté milks the goats and sheep! Why does he not make the Devil tell us how the brilliante conquete managed her Dairy?"

Hill's tirade against French translators is followed by a no less envenomed attack on French critics. They base their comments, he alleges, on inadequate translations, speak dogmatically on what they do not understand and are inclined to attribute praise of Milton to national prejudice.

His survey of engraved portraits of Milton selects William Faithorne's (1670) as the best and condemns many others. He appends a selection of adverse criticism and mentions a copy of the 1674 edition of *Paradise Lost* in which the following lines were written in a contemporary hand:

> Milton his clubb hath cast at Paradise
> blind in his fancy as hee's in his eyes
> what need we all this bable of the spheres
> had right been don, he should have lost his ears
> this book shall nere procure him a good fame
> Eikonoclastes doth record his shame.

Hill's copious notes occupy 240 pages of closely-written script; I shall confine comment to a few in which we encounter the doctor in his legitimate role of natural scientist.

Referring to the ancient River Adonis which yearly "Ran purple to the sea, supposed with blood" (Bk I, 451), Hill suggests "the dust or farina of the flowers of the Juniper, Pine and Fir" may give the water its reddish tinge. He will not have it that Empedocles leaped into the flames of Mount Etna (III, 471); it is more likely that in his quest for knowledge the philosopher stood too close to the mouth of the erupting volcano and was suffocated.

The concept of the Phoenix derives from the date tree which stirs Hill's botanical imagination. "It is indeed not to be wondered at, that a tree so singular in its Nature should supply a subject for ingenious fiction. A tree which grows and flourishes only in the burning sands and burning winds of the torrid Zone; which retains its vigour and fruitfulness for Ages; And at length, when rather satiated with life than worn down by time, burns and dies, that a youthful Successor may spring up from its aromatic ashes, to bloom like the parent plant, and to run through an equally protracted period of Existence".

"... Greedily they plucked/The fruitage fair to sight, like that which grew /Neer that bituminous Lake where Sodom flam's " (X 560). The reference, Hill points out, is to the Poma Sodomitica also called Mala insana or Mad Apples. They abound about Jerico not far from the Dead Sea. They are attacked by an insect which turns the inside to dust leaving the skin entire and of a beautiful colour.

The line "Conspicious with three listed Colours gay" (XI 866) leads Hill to mention that Isaac Newton's analysis of light into seven colours being unknown to Milton he accepts Aristotle's scheme.

Hill devotes a lengthy passage to Milton's lines on his blindness:

> So thick a Drop serene hath quench't their orbs,
> Or dim Suffusion veil'd (III 25).

He explains that the Gutta serena or Amaurosis "called here a Drop serene, is a total extinction of Sight, without any perceptible injury of the form or constitution of the Eye, which still retains its brightness and transparency ..." The causes of the disease "are of too subtile a nature for discovery". The older explanation of "a cold, transparent watery humour that dropped upon the Optic Nerve and destroyed its function" is no longer tenable but it may be the result of "a paralytic affection of the retina", a disease of the brain or pressure on the optic nerves.

The diagnosis of Milton's blindness remains uncertain; modern discussants add chronic glaucoma and detached retina to the disorders mentioned as possible causes by Dr Hill[10]

"Erinensis", a London journal's Dublin correspondent, encountered Dr Hill at a social occasion in Mercer's Hospital where, in the 1820s, Hill then in his eighties retained his position as physician and governor. Erinensis was a satirist who liked to lampoon Dublin doctors and their institutions but his portrait of Edward Hill may be genuine enough.

> By accident he was dressed in the fashion; his coat, to the cut of which he has inviolably adhered for sixty years, presenting then as great a space between the hip buttons, as the most "exquisite" of his neighbours. He talked of the Greek and Arabian lights of medicine, of Rhazes and Avicenna ... and on entering the room, I thought that one of the figures of Hogarth's "Examination at Surgeon's Hall" had descended from the wall, to converse with us on the topics of his day.[11]

Hill appeared to enjoy himself and Erinensis felt it must be a consolation to the physician's juniors, with the prospect of old age still remote, "to behold successive cargoes of everything on the board descend into the hold of an octogenarian vessel that had sailed in safety across the quicksands of all the climacterics, and whose timbers still promised to withstand the assaults of many another gale".

A survivor from the eighteenth century, Hill lived until 1830, by which time Robert Graves, William Stokes and Dominic Corrigan had taken leadership in Dublin medicine. His anachronistic presence would have lacked authority in the face of innovations like the stethoscope. He must not be judged beside the young stalwarts of the "golden age" of Irish medicine. He belongs to another era and illustrates a curious symbiosis involving medicine and literature; he stands alongside Paul Hiffernan, Oliver Goldsmith and Sylvester O'Halloran in a line continued by Robert Richard Madden, Sir William Wilde and George Sigerson in the nineteenth century.

Hill genuinely attempted to improve the Dublin medical school. He was outsmarted in the physic garden affair but his endeavours in this regard should be viewed in the wider context of Irish horticulture. In the last quarter of the eighteenth century according to Charles Nelson,[12] "botany and horticulture were still slumbering here, and it was Edward Hill who stirred the sleeping beauty". His Miltonic manuscript is a polemical tour de force; whether it possesses intrinsic merit is a question to address to literary scholars who seem to have passed it by.

ACKNOWLEDGEMENTS

I am indebted to the Board of Trinity College, Dublin, for permission to quote from Hill's manuscript and to reproduce the title-page of the Catalogue. The portrait of Edward Hill is included by courtesy of the Royal College of Physicians of Ireland. Vincent Kinane permitted access to his unpublished work on the Dublin University Press and Mary O'Doherty helped me in many ways.

REFERENCES

1.   Kirkpatrick T P C, *History of the Medical School in Trinity College Dublin.* Dublin: Hanna and Neale, 1912

2.   Widdess J D H, *A History of the Royal College of Physicians of Ireland.* Edinburgh: Livingstone, 1963

3.   Hill E, *An Address to the Students of Physic.* Dublin, 1803

4.   Kinane V, *The Dublin University Press in the Eighteenth Century.* Thesis submitted for Fellowship of the Library Association of Ireland, 1981

5.   *Dr Hill's Library: A Catalogue.* Dublin, 1816

6.   Bell R, "Life of John Milton", pp 251-256 in *Eminent Literary and Scientific Men, 1.* London: Longman, 1839

7.   Lyons J B, *Scholar & Sceptic.* Dublin: Glendale Press, 1986

8.   TCD Ms 629. 1=5

9.   Todd H J ed, *The Poetical Works of John Milton,* seven vols. Second ed, with verbal index to the whole of Milton's poetry. London: Law and Gilbert, 1809

10.   Brown E G, *Milton's Blindness.* New York, 1934

11.   Fallon M, *The Sketches of Erinensis.* London: Skilton and Shaw, 1979

12.   Nelson E C. "Botany, Medicine and Politics in Eighteenth Century Dublin". *Moorea,* **6**, pp 33-44, 1987

"SECRET NOSTRUMS" Aspects of the Development of Patent and Proprietary Medicines

Terence D Turner

The granting of a royal commercial monopoly was at one time a matter of both pleasure and personal profit to the sovereign. Queen Elizabeth I so abused the system that towards the end of her reign public discontent forced her to modify her "gifting" and her successor James I was expected to do the same.[1]

Unfortunately the abuse continued until the regulation of such grants came into the hands of parliament under the Statute of Monopolies which was passed in 1624. This statute limited the period of privilege to fourteen years although a further application could be made for letters patent renewal.

Until approximately 1720 the administration of this Act did not require specifications of either processes or formula as part of the patent submission. It was considered that those employed in the manufacture of the patented products would acquire knowledge and skills and by changing their jobs or becoming self employed they would negate any contrived monopoly.

During the reign of Queen Anne the situation changed and there were new requirements for specifications to be filed before letters patent were issued. This included medicinal products, but was not rigorously applied. It was recognised that the therapeutic effect of a medicine could be attributed not only to the activity of its ingredients but also to the placebic contribution of the presentation and the contrived mystery surrounding the product. To identify the precise formula in a specification would have destroyed this mystery and eventually ruined the sale and allowed others to copy the remedy and, where the ingredients were obtainable, to compound it themselves.

In effect the term "patent medicines" became a contradictory description of "secret remedies". The complexity of their formulation frequently defied analysis and although competitors could detect the major active constituents the originator could claim that only he knew the complete formula and secret of their blending. By the mid-eighteenth century there were some hundreds of patent medicines which could be purchased by the man in the street. Their composition was made more complex by the availability of new exotic plants that had come from overseas and of new chemical remedies which had originated with Paracelsus and subsequently developed. Polypharmaceuticals abounded, composed of many ingredients to cover all possible clinical conditions.

The multitude of remedies had little justification for their existence other than a wish on the part of the inventor and producer to make a financial profit and on the part of the sick person to recover health. The general popular trend towards self-medication had to some degree been forced upon the community by the refusal of the London College of Physicians to expand the number of practitioners on their register, although it was estimated that there were over 1300 serious cases of illness per day for every member of the college. Thus the public sought their treatment from the hands of well meaning empirics and unscrupulous quacks, the latter having no legal or moral restraint in suggesting a new medicine.

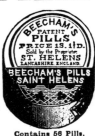

LARGEST SALES! QUICKEST TURNOVER!

WORTH A GUINEA A BOX.

BEECHAM'S ✣ PILLS

FOR ALL

Bilious and Nervous Disorders,

Sick Headache, Constipation,

Wind and Pains in Stomach, Impaired Digestion,

Disordered Liver, and Female Ailments.

The Sale now EXCEEDS SIX MILLION BOXES per annum.

Druggists will find BEECHAM'S PILLS the MOST SALEABLE Patent Medicine in the Market.

Contains 56 Pills.

BEECHAM'S COUGH PILLS

STAND UNRIVALLED FOR

Coughs, Asthma, Bronchial Affections, Hoarseness, &c., &c.

In Boxes, 1s. 1½d. and 2s. 9d. each, with full directions.

BEECHAM'S TOOTH PASTE

RECOMMENDS ITSELF.

It is Efficacious, Economical, Cleanses the Teeth, Perfumes the Breath, and is a Reliable and Pleasant Dentifrice.

In Collapsible Tubes, of all Druggists, ONE SHILLING each.

Home Retailers of BEECHAM'S PILLS desirous of exhibiting Show Cards or Dummies, and wishful to have a good supply of Handbills (various sizes and colours, with name and address at foot), Oracles, Puzzles, &c., should apply to the Proprietor—

THOMAS BEECHAM, ST. HELENS, LANCASHIRE.

44. Advertisement for Beecham's Pills in *The Chemist and Druggist, 28 July 1906*

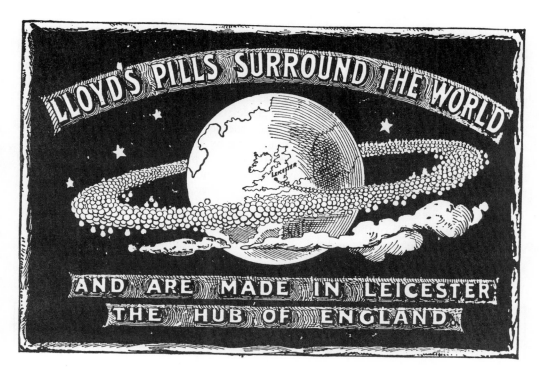

45. Advertisement for Lloyd's Pills from *Chemist and Druggist 1905*

Another factor which contributed to the demand for patent medicine was the physicians' charges which were extortionate and those of the apothecaries who were very expensive. For example, a Mr Dolby of Ludgate Hill was treated by an apothecary for four days at a cost £2..17..0 per day. In contrast a bottle of Fryar's balsam cost 1/- which was then the monetary equivalent of a day's wage.

Nostrum promotion was therefore greater in the eighteenth century than at any other time. If one wished to substantially increase an income a nostrum was discovered, advertisements printed, a number of cases cited, cures attested, a patent procured and a pamphlet published. In the early eighteenth century the nostrums would be sold at inns and taverns. Later the sales changed to the booksellers, druggists, apothecaries and frequently doctor inventors. As the patentees died or patents lapsed the more popular products became "secret recipes" in the hands of a small number of manufacturers and distributors. Some products remained within a family. Careful control of distribution and personal validation by a successor of the inventor was often sufficient to prevent them falling into the hands of the new "wholesalers". The self styled "Sir" John Hill - a title which he justified on the strength of an award of the Order of Vasca from the King of Sweden for a 26 volume work on *The Vegetable System* - was better known in England for his *Family Herbal* and his patent medicine "Hill's Pectoral Balsam". When he died in 1775 his wife maintained control by authenticating each bottle by signing her name on the label with red ink "thus avoiding false copies".

In 1785 there were 130 registered patent medicines; by 1802 these had increased to 550 and it can be assumed that there was a large number of other non-official remedies in circulation.[2] The invention of the paper making machine in 1798 and the discovery of the principle of lithography at approximately the same time resulted in an increase in the availability of pamphlets and of newspaper advertising and the appearance of printed medicine labels made the public more aware of a medicine's claimed properties and thus further increased its popularity. It is estimated that by 1895 one manufacturer had sold 2,519,856 boxes of his sugar coated pills and Beecham's pills were said to have been sold at the rate of one million pills for each day of the week including Sundays, with an annual turnover in the 1890's of £360,000.[3]

The first medicines to obtain letters patent are shown in Table 1.[4] These and other patents granted in the first half of the eighteenth century contribute to our understanding of the developments of the products and the response of the community.

Epsom salts and Stoughton's Elixir are two preparations which illustrate the contrast which existed in origin, content and usage.

Table 1. Early Patent Medicines			
Epsom Salts	Nehemiah Grew	1698	No 354
"Sal Oleum Volatile"	Timothy Byfield	1711	No 388
Stoughtons Elixir	Richard Stoughton	1712	No 390
Hoopers Female Pills	John Hooper	1743	No 592
Turlingtons Balsam	Robert Turlington	1744	No 596
Toothache Tincture	Thomas Greenhough	1744	No 599

Epsom Salts

It is questionable whether naturally occurring magnesium sulphate produced by evaporation of the spring water from Epsom can be considered as a proprietary medicine but it cannot be ignored as one of the first medicinal compounds to be the subject of a patent. In 1698 this "hydragogue cathartic" was granted letters patent by William III who expressed a willingness to "cherish and encourage all lawdable endeavours and designs of such of our subjects who have .... found out useful and profitable arts, mysteries and inventions". The patentee was Nehemiah Grew, a London physician, who was Secretary of the Royal Society and to which he had presented a treatise *On the Bitter Cathartic Salt of the Epsom Waters*.[1]

Unfortunately the granting of a patent did not bring the security of rights of ownership which it suggests, indeed it frequently stimulated others into producing direct copies or products of similar composition or activity.

Stoughton's Elixir

Dr Richard Stoughton's greatest claim to fame is as the inventor of "Elixir Magnum Stomachium" or the "Great Cordial Elixir".[5] Although the Elixir was not patented until 1712 it was being marketed around 1690 and by 1708 Stoughton announced in a newspaper advertisement that many of his customers were taking 40 to 50 bottles a year and that it was available from all coffee house and booksellers in and about London.

The patent granted by Queen Anne described the Elixir as "A new and most useful and Restorative Cordial and medicine ...... gained an Universal Esteem throughout our Kingdome of Great Britain and Ireland and likewise in many Forreiyn Parts".

The patent claimed that it contained 22 ingredients "unknown to any other one but me". Its chief constituents would appear to have been Gentian, Serpentary, Orange Peel, Cardamon and Rhubarb. Other botanicals may have been included and the French *Codex Medicamentaurius* of 1818 gave a formula for Tincture Amara, "dicta vulgo Elixirium Doctoris Stoughton" which included wormwood, cascarilla and aloes.

It was claimed as a remedy for all distemper of the stomach and the recommended dosage was "Fifty or sixty drops ... more or less as you please, taken in a glass of Spring Water, Beer, Ale, Tea, Canary Cyder, White Wine, with or without sugar, a dram of Brandy as often as you please but especially in the morning fasting".

As with other nostrums of the period the broadside claims were as wide as the recommended posology.

Richard Stoughton's patent was left to his wife and thereafter to his two sons and it expired in 1726, fourteen years after being granted. As with many of the proprietary medicines of that period the ingredients were eventually revealed in pharmacopoeias and other formularies, and Stoughton's Elixir was still included in the 1953 edition of *Pharmaceutical Formulae*.[6] It is difficult to identify a proprietary product or indeed an ethically approved drug currently on the drug market which will still be available in the year 2,251, a period equivalent to that survived by Stoughton's Elixir throughout the reigns of fourteen kings and queens of Great Britain.

Scots Pills

One of the oldest patent medicines was "Anderson's Scots Pills". They were on sale in 1630's and still available in 1916. They were available from Patrick Anderson, a doctor, who was reputed to have been physician to Charles I. In 1635 he published his text *Grana Angelica*, a treatise in Latin describing the virtues of his pill.[7]

Anderson's Scots Pill gained respectability with age but it was fully justified as a purgative, each of the major components Aloe and Colocynth being renowned emetics.

GRANA ANGELICA
OR, THE TRUE
SCOTS PILLS.

Left to Posterity by Dr. PATRICK ANDERSON of Edinburgh, Physician to
His Majesty K. Ch. I. and constantly used as his Ordinary Physick by K. Ch. II.
Are Faithfully prepared Only by I. INGLISH from Edinburgh,
Now living at the Unicorn over-against the Watch-house near the May-Pole in the Strand, London.
~By Her MAJESTIES Authority.

Amongst the most eminent Physicians of this Age, the late famous Doctor ANDERSON is most deservedly to be esteemed: For he spared
no Travel nor Study that might be serviceable to the Diseased of his Country; and returning from his Travels, with a Mind fully enriched,
amongst other Things, he brought from Venice this inestimable Jewel, whose Virtues and Uses are these:
I. They exceedingly comfort and strengthen the Stomach; they restore the lost Appetite, they purge Choler and Melancholy, but chiefly Phlegm
and waterish Matter: They cleanse the same of all putrid, gross and thick Humours, they comfort the Intrails, open Obstructions, and disperse all
the Pain of these Places.
II. They strengthen the Head and all the Senses, but chiefly those of Hearing and Sight, whose Weakness and Pain they remove; they help the
Giddiness thereof, and the Megrim: And as they comfort and purge the Stomach, so they do the like both to Head and Heart; and have this excellent Faculty, That being mix'd with other Physick, they correct its Malignity, and make it unhurtful to the Stomach; and are therefore to be preferred to all other gentle and easie Medicines.
III. They are wonderfully helpful to all Diseases of the Womb, and all other Maladies belonging to Women, that proceed from Coldness, by Chance,
or Constitution; For they safely and easily purge and empty the Belly, without Pain or Gripings, and carry out by their proper Passages all those vicious Humours, and other Dregs, that are stopped in a Woman after her Delivery: And they much help Barrenness that proceedeth from Unclean-
ness of the Womb, and cleanse Women from their White Flux, and so fitteth and enableth them for Conception. Also they may be taken by Women with Child, for yielding them Ease in their Bellies gently, without any hazard of miscarrying at all, one every Night before Supper.
IV. They kill and choke all Worms that are bred in the Wombs of Children, Big-bellied Women that are bound in the Belly, and of Men; Yea,
not any Body, that frequently useth these Pills, can breed Worms at all.

46. Advertisement for Anderson's Scots Pills.

The accolade of acceptability was the inclusion in the *Codex Pharmacopée Francaise*[8] of 1839 of Pilules Ecossaises, and as reported in the 1899 edition of *Pharmaceutical Formulae*, the medicine was represented in the British Pharmacopoeia as Pilulae Aloe et Myrrhai. Most proprietary medicines were the subject of fraudulent imitators but Anderson's pills were exceptional in being counterfeited by Isabella Inglish who, although denounced by Edinburgh Town Council in 1690, continued to sell "true Scots Pills". Indeed both Anderson's and Inglish's Scots Pills were rivals for more than 150 years and only disappeared from the catalogue of Raimee Clark & Co in 1916.

Morison's Pills

James Morison named his product the "Vegetable Universal Medicine" and postulated a Hygeian canon in which the blood controls everything and all disease comes from impurities within it; these must be purged by vegetables and it was said to be impossible to purge too much.

The pill has been given various formulations but it was not dissimilar to Anderson's pills in containing the traditional natural product cathartics.[9] They were produced as a No 1 and No 2 presentation. The dosage was remarkable, the 1830's brochure recommends that "No 1 and 2 are both aperient and purgative and may be used indiscriminately, but experience has proved that No 2 is the most efficacious in subduing many diseases, in fevers of all kinds, inflammation, asthma, smallpox, measles, gout, colic, and cancer. In all violent diseases or pain it is necessary to take one dose of No 1 today, the same of No 2 tomorrow and repeat No 2 the next day increasing the dose by one pill every third day." It is not surprising that patients took very large numbers of pills and for example a London grocer was reported as taking 18,000 pills. Morison claimed "... the larger the dose ... the easier they act and do more good". Not all proprietary products were to be as successful in the approach to selling as Morison's . He chose to concentrate on three promotional aspects: first, a single cause and a single cure for all diseases. Second, the ignorance and evil of the medical profession and thirdly continuous publicity through pamphlets and broadsheets. The success of his venture and the opportunistic nature of the man combined with his distrust of the medical profession resulted in his building in 1828 the "British College of Health". From this imposing building he carried out an active campaign against doctors, he produced *Hygeian Illustrations* and the *Hygeist Journal* and the title page of *Morisonia* proclaimed "The Old Medical Science is completely wrong".

Between 1834 and 1836 a number of deaths were attributed to Morison's pills. Public criticism was aroused and continued even after Morison's death in 1842 when the business of the British College of Health was passed to his two sons. On the principle that bad publicity is better than none at all, the product was kept before the public eye and marketed in both USA and the rest of Europe, and in the 1850's chemists and druggists began to stock and distribute the pills. It is probable that Morison's pills and his marketing approach were one of the earliest successful examples of applied sales psychology and certainly one of the first instances of the technique being used on a proprietary medicine.

The Stamp Act

In the last quarter of the eighteenth century the Chancellor, Lord Cavendish, was forced to impose a tax on a variety of merchandise and also on servants, mules, carriages, dogs, clocks, watches and of course medicines. This "temporary" tax of 1783 lasted 158 years until 1941.[10]

The Stamp Act and the associated licensing of sellers and premises had a marked effect upon the sale and distribution of patent and proprietary medicines. The first Act of 1783 was directed at the immediate receipt of monies by the Treasury. It required that Vendors and Sellers of medicines in Great Britain should possess an annual licence to sell. The cost of the licence was £1 in London, Westminster and the penny postal area, elsewhere was reduced to 5/- per annum. "Any person who had been an apprentice to a Surgeon, Apothecary, Druggist or Chymist was exempt as also were commissioned surgeons in the Army or Navy and those who had maintained a premises for the sole sale of medicines and drugs for three years prior to the Act."

In addition to the annual licence individual medicines were taxed and duty was payable at 3d for a face value of 2s 6d or less, 6d for the value of 2s 6d to 5s and 1s for values exceeding 5s. The vendors had to send their wrappers or covers or labels with the correct amount of tax to the Commissioners of Stamps and these were returned suitably franked. Fraud in terms of counterfeit stamps or re-use of wrappers was vigorously controlled through common informers who shared the fines equally with the Crown.

The entire act was considered to be a tax on the sick and arguments put forward at that time have been repeated recently in the proposed application of charges for services and medicaments within the National Health Service.

Public pressure required amendments to be made and in 1785 the 1783 Act was repealed and replaced by a new act which differed primarily in exempting certain classes of medicines, in particular those specified in the first and second "Books of Rates" initiated in 1660[10] which were import duties upon almost all materials used by Spicers, Druggists and Apothecaries.

Also exempted were preparations sold by exempted persons provided that the "Properties, Qualities, Virtues and Efficacies are *known, admitted and approved* in the prevention or treatment of human ailments". This exemption only applied to remedies where there was no claim to exclusive right either in manufacturing or distribution; thus patent medicines were excluded.

In 1786 a further act included perfumes and related products under a separate annual licence to deal in perfumery. In 1802 the 1785 Act was repealed and a more definitive product description was passed. It stated that "upon every packet, box, bottle or other inclosure containing any drugs, herbs, waters, essences, tincture, powders or other preparations or compositions whatsoever used or applied externally there must be a duty stamp affixed."

Modifying Acts such as that of 1803 and new acts such as those of 1804, 1812, 1815 and 1833 changed the duties payable and brought in all medicines for which proprietary rights were claimed or advertised. Lozenges and mineral waters were the subject of particular attention in 1812, 1815 and 1833.

The continuing "tax on sickness" on both licence to sell and individual proprietary items did not appear to discourage the general public from the on-going commitment to self-medication, indeed the "stamp" with its "official label design" gave a certain accreditation to the medicine and proprietors sought to develop the false concept that the addition of the Government Stamp indicated a Commission approval of its quality and efficacy. Stamps purchased to affix to their products were allowed to have the proprietor's name printed upon them. This was sometimes accompanied by a spurious claim which the unsuspecting customer would accept as having the authority of the Crown. The practice became so widely spread that in 1885 it was ordered that the stamp should include the words "No Government Guarantee". Even so the practice of including "official" style labelling with illustrations of national and international medallions and medals continued to give an "up market" image to many proprietaries for many years.

The difficulty of distinguishing medicine and remedy caused the Customs and Excise to rule in 1915 that "where the name of an ailment is mentioned on a label duty is required but where only the organ to be treated is mentioned no duty is levied". Thus:

DUTY REQUIRED	NO DUTY REQUIRED
Cough Mixture Liver Tonic Corn Paint Headache Powder	Chest Mixture Liver Mixture Toe Paint Head Powder

There is no doubt that the financial yield to Government from this tax was significant. In the early 1900's the licence holders paying 5s numbered 43,156 and yielded £10,791 duty. In 1908 the numbers of excise stamps issued was 41,757,575 made up of 33 million at 1 1/2d, 7 1/2 million at 3d and 1 million at 6d giving an excise duty yield of £30,000. Whilst this is a significant amount it is worth noting that in the same period the turnover of Beecham's pills grossed £360,000 per annum.

The distinction between patent and proprietary medicines was now more difficult to identify than previously. The group of products which had been declared exempt from the tax in 1785 second Stamp Act were those which were "known admitted and approved" products for which no proprietary claims were made by the seller. This meant that if a new product was produced by a pharmacist and could be shown to meet this requirement no tax would be levied. Sir William Glyn Jones sought to have this position clarified in the courts, using as an example Ammoniated Tincture of Quinine of the *British Pharmacopoeia* labelled "a well known and highly recommended remedy for influenza and colds". A divisional court confirmed the validity of this product exemption by virtue of it being a Pharmacopoeial preparation without proprietary claims. This ruling resulted in pharmacists inserting their formula for a medicine in an "admitted book of reference" and the publication of *The Pharmaceutical Journal of Formulary* in 1898 fulfilled the requirements.[8]

No duty was now payable on such medicines and by comparison with taxable proprietaries the preparations were not only cheaper but carried the professional guarantee of the compounder. This had a marked effect on the proprietary market. Similar products to those newly obtainable from the pharmacist disappeared. A greater public sensitivity to the content of medicines was aroused and demands made that all proprietary medicines should compulsorily disclose their formula. Many proposals to produce legislation to enforce this requirement were made but vested interests succeeded in blocking the necessary parliamentary action. The Select Committee on Patent Medicines in its report in the *Lancet* in September 1914 observed that " ... the vendors of patent and proprietary medicines can practically do what they like so long as they keep outside the bounds of gross and obvious impropriety ..."[11]

It is an unsavoury truth that many did press these boundaries of propriety very close and it was not until the passage of the Pharmacy and Medicine Act of 1941 that disclosure of active ingredients was enforced. The stamp taxation was discontinued to be replaced by Purchase Tax. Other changes in legislation on advertising and treatment claims have modified the proprietary medicine market[12] and every product must declare its composition and have its medical claims validated by the Commission on Safety of Medicines. It is however interesting to reflect that certain potent herbal medicines sold in the reign of Elizabeth I are still available to the general public who have even less awareness of their quality and efficacy than their forefathers. These would appear to be the last of the "secret nostrums" and will surely be eventually controlled to prevent the possible exploitation of the sick and innocent.

REFERENCES

1.   Wooton A C, *Chronicles of Pharmacy*. London, 1910. Vol 2, p 168

2.   *Chemist and Druggist*. 1936, Special Issue, p 758

3.   Propretaries of other days. *Chem Drugg*, June 1927, p 835

4.   *Codex Pharmacopee Française*. Paris, 1839, p 447

5.   Young J H, *The Toadstool Millionaires*. New Jersey, Princeton University Press, 1961, p 7

6.   Ibid. 1953, p 173

7.   Jackson W A, Grana Angelica. *Pharm Hist*, 1987, **17**, 2-5

8.   "Pharmaceutical Formulae". *The Chemist and Druggist*, 1898, p 575

9.   Helfand W H, *Trans Brit Soc Hist Pharm*. 1974, **1**.3. p 101

10. Matthews L G, The Medicine Stamp Acts of Great Britain. *Pharm Historian*, 1986, **16,** p 25

11. *The Lancet*: Report of the Select Committee on Patent Medicines. Sept 5, 1914, p 653

12. Chapman H E, Proprietary Medicines - The Present Position. *Pharm J*, 1955, **175,** p 207

THE NINETEENTH CENTURY DOMESTIC MEDICINE CHEST

Anne Young

"A judicious and discerning public have long experienced, and repeatedly acknowledged, the inestimable advantages derived from a portable dispensary".

Addressed to the literate and monied classes this opening sentence from *Cox's Companion to the Family Medicine Chest*, the new edition of 1824,[1] suggests that by this date domestic medicine chests were well established at least among the "carriage trade". The gentry, when living in their country houses, needed a supply of medicines readily to hand in view of the time it would have taken to get medical help. Such people too would have been expected to deal with illness in their employees and in the poor of the neighbourhood, as would the local clergymen.

Domestic medicine chests, having evolved from those used by armies[2] and the travelling aristocracy, were common on the Continent from the seventeenth century as plague remedies were required by law to be kept in the home.[3] In this country, however, even eighteenth century examples are rare. Those that have survived are small, custom built, wooden or fish skin covered boxes, velvet lined, and holding six to eight round bottles. Then, in the last decade of the eighteenth century they became very much commoner, almost "mass produced". By 1808 they were available in a multitude of styles. These nineteenth century chests are large, beautifully made in mahogany, and filled with twenty or so bottles, square or rectangular in section. They also contain apparatus for compounding medicaments.

It is not possible to gather much information from the relatively few chests that appear for sale as contemporary contents are frequently lacking or they have been over-enthusiastically restored. Fortunately, there is a large number - 463 to be precise - in the Wellcome Collection. Few are on view but detailed catalogue cards are available[4] and Table 1 summarises the collection.

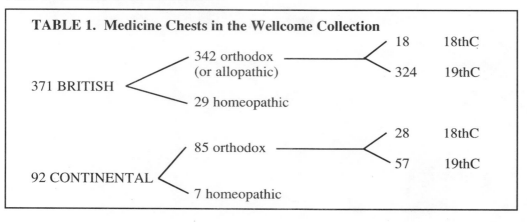

TABLE 1. Medicine Chests in the Wellcome Collection

371 BRITISH
- 342 orthodox (or allopathic)
  - 18 — 18thC
  - 324 — 19thC
- 29 homeopathic

92 CONTINENTAL
- 85 orthodox
  - 28 — 18thC
  - 57 — 19thC
- 7 homeopathic

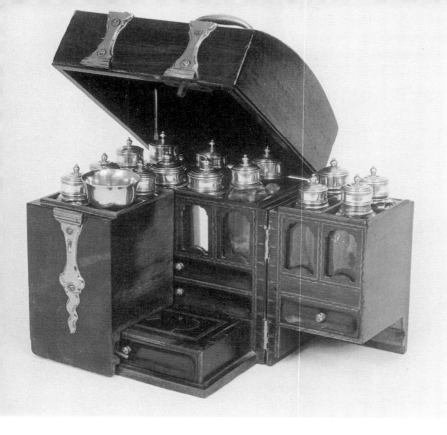

47. (Left) Brass bound coromandel chest with silver fittings. Continental c1720. Note silver funnel on left and round silver powder container.

48. (Below) Left: English mahogany chest with silver fittings. c1750. Right: Fish-skin covered chest with brass lock and feet. English c1780. Note the more usual round bottles of 18th century chests. Glass medicine funnel in foreground.

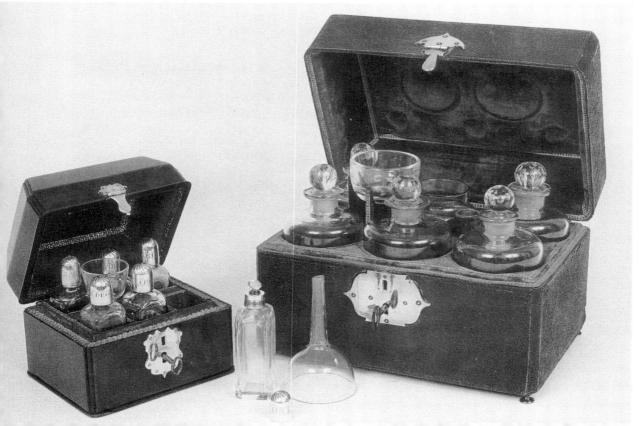

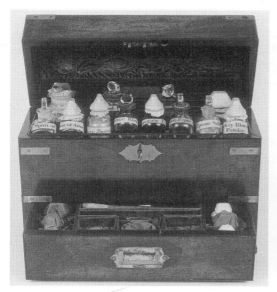

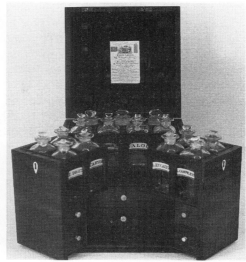

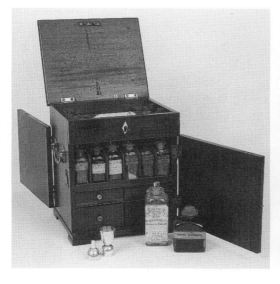

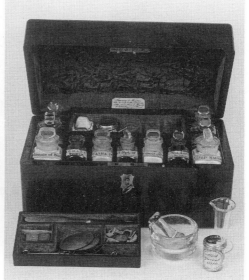

49. (Top left). Mahogany brass bound chest. Trunk opening style c1840.

50. (Bottom left). "Duke of York" style mahogany chest c1820. In foreground, one of the four tall bottles from main compartment; also one of six small bottles from rear of chest.

51. (Top right). "Raj-style" chest. Mahogany. c1850. *(Courtesy of Christopher Sykes Antiques, Woburn).*

52. (Bottom right). Rosewood chest with "nesting drawers" c1840. Tray contains scales, weights and spatula, mortar and pestle, silver capped jar and measuring glass.

Commonest amongst the British chests, because fashionable both at the turn of the century and again in the second half of the nineteenth century,[5] are those which open like a trunk with a rising lid and a drawer at the base. (Illustration 49) A brass retaining rod ensures that the drawer cannot be opened once the chest is closed and locked. Variations include a type where the drawer is replaced by nesting trays in the body of the chest.(Illustration 52) A popular style at the turn of the century was the so-called "Duke of York"[6] with rising lid and doors front and back.(Illustration 50) Again brass levers ensure that the doors cannot be opened once the lid is down and the chest locked. A rarer style produced at this time has a rising lid and winged doors. The bottles are housed in the central part, and in the doors, behind fenestrated wooden partitions. The shape of the fenestrations reminds me of Indian architecture, and I therefore call this the "Raj style" (Illustration 51)

Perhaps the most attractive of all, though rarer still, are those made in imitation of spice cupboards with bottles and accessories concealed behind false drawer panels. (Illustration 53)

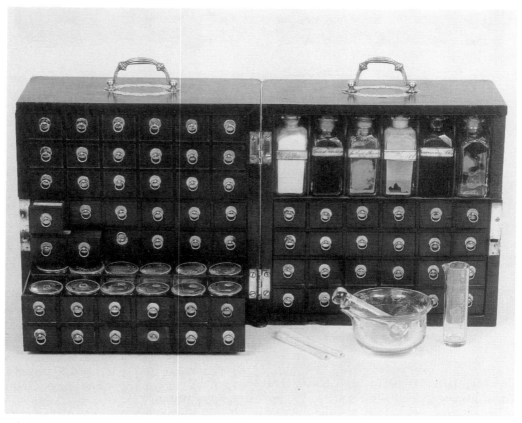

53. English mahogany chest with silver carrying handles c1760. The chest opens to reveal various sized drawers and a sliding panel (removed) covering a set of jars. Pestle and mortar, a measuring glass and 2 ivory enema nozzles are in the foreground.

In the early nineteenth century the trunk-like boxes appear to have been supplanted for a time by those which open like a double fronted cupboard, the doors holding galleries of bottles (Illustration 54). The larger of these have four to six bottles at the back, concealed by a sliding panel. Again the rear compartment cannot be opened once the chest is locked, demonstrating the skill of the cabinet makers. Although frequently called "poison compartments", the bottles at the back hold innocuous substances like tartaric acid and bicarbonate of soda. Table 2 summarises the cabinet styles of the 371 British chests in the Wellcome Collection. 7.5% of the collection are individually styled and of unusual form, and it is these that are now particularly popular with collectors.

Table 2. Cabinet Styles

%	STYLE	FASHIONABLE PERIOD
57%	TRUNK with rising lid	Late 18C Mid -late 19thC
17%	"DUKE OF YORK" rising lid, doors front and rear	Late 18th - early 19thC
13%	CUPBOARD with winged doors	First half 19thC
4%	"RAJ" rising lid and winged doors	Late 18th - early 19thC
1.5%	"SPICE CUPBOARD"	Turn 18thC

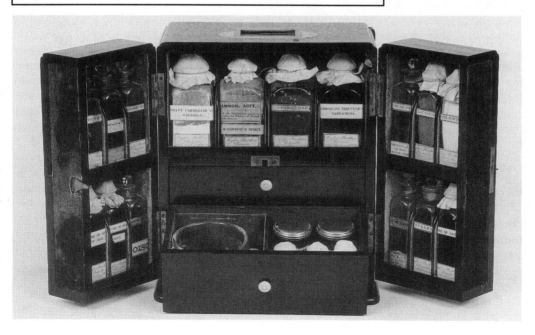

54. (Below) Mahogany chest, "cupboard" style. c1860.

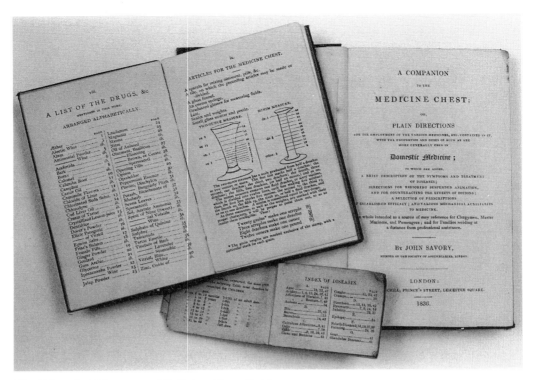

55. (Above). 19th century Medicine Chest Guides.

The chests were made by those specialist cabinet makers responsible for tea caddies, liquor boxes, dressing chests, etc and advertised by the chemists and druggists who fitted them out.[7] Doctors who wrote for the lay public recommended their use and prominent amongst them was the enterprising Dr Richard Reece. He not only wrote a *Medical Guide* and *A Practical Dictionary of Domestic Medicine*[8] but also sold chests and medicines at his "MEDICAL AND CHYMICAL HALL" at 170 Piccadilly. There is a fine mahogany Reece chest on view at the Wellcome Galleries in the Science Museum, but Reece also catered for "the lower orders and impoverished clergymen" (sic) by offering "economical chests of oak or deal fitted with corked black bottles". (The flint glass bottles in the chests for the wealthy have ground glass stoppers).

A list has been made of the labels on the bottles in the Wellcome chests[9] and this shows that about half were fitted by London chemists and druggists, e g Savory, later Savory & Moore; Cooke, later Godfrey & Cooke; and Peter Squire, who in 1837 became the first chemist and druggist, as opposed to apothecary, to be granted the Royal Warrant.[10] The remainder have bottles supplied by chemists in towns all over the United Kingdom. Several bear labels from further afield - France, America, India - a piquant reminder of our travelling and Empire-building forebears.

As it is impossible to be certain that the chest contents are contemporary, information on the drugs and apparatus originally supplied can best be gathered from the many Medicine

Chest Guides which were published.(Illustration 55) A few were sold with the chests,[11] but the majority were sold separately. All are now scarce, and when found, often in a very tattered state. All include lists of the drugs and apparatus to be kept in the chest,[12] an explanation of apothecary weights and measures,[13] and tables on adjustment of dosage according to age.[14] All go on to list the various drugs, ointments, etc, giving under each their properties and the indications for their use.[15] The longer guides have, in addition, sections on diseases and their treatment,[16] all reflecting the orthodox medical practice of the time. Most sound a note of caution. Savory[17] for example wrote - "It is, however, earnestly recommended not to place too much confidence on books of Domestic Medicine, especially in such cases as are of a serious nature, but always to have recourse to the advice of an able physician as early as it can be obtained".

The apparatus in the chests is fitted into beautifully tailored compartments in a standardised way. Scales, weights, measuring glass, mortar and pestle, are present even in small chests. Some also have a pill tile, spatula, plaster iron, and caustic-stick. A probang (a flexible stick "to dislodge that which is stuck in the gullet"), plasters or "Court plaister" and "Gold-beaters' skin" are rarer finds. Occasionally leech-tubes are present, leeches being commonly used on a "self-help" basis. Maw's *Guide* advertises "Improved Leech Appliers ... of wire gauze, in four sizes, 1/6d each, of Glass 6d each".[18]

Turning now to the drugs, whereas eighteenth century chests contain a handful of simple restoratives (eg Sal Volatile, Lavender drops, Hartshorn), nineteenth century chests may contain 40 or more including calomel, tartar emetic (an antimony preparation), and opium. J.K. Crellin made a detailed study of the drugs in the Wellcome chests[19] and concluded that three main therapeutic categories - purgatives, stimulants and preparations for external application - are always well represented. Other categories - emetics, diaphoretics, pain killers, fever remedies and anti-convulsants - are represented by only one or two items for each category, even in the largest chests.

In chests I have studied antacids have featured and these include Calcined Magnesia, Natron (Sodium Carbonate), Testaceous Powder prepared from crushed oyster shells, and the expensive Gascoign's Balls, a mixture of pounded crabs claws, pearls, red coral and Oriental Bezoar. It is notable that although proprietary preparations were legion in the nineteenth century, few appeared in the chest contents lists apart from the ubiquitous Dover's , James' and Gregory's powders which, along with one or two others, appear to have been awarded generic status. The ingredients of the handwritten family receipt books such as herbs, snail juice and other animal products do not appear either.

In this climate where the approach to illness - any illness - was to get rid of it either upwards with emetics, downwards with purgatives, or outwards by sweating it out with diaphoretics (the body further assaulted by blistering and the removal of pints of blood) it is not surprising that the much gentler homeopathic approach was welcomed. Brought to this country in 1820 by Dr Frederick Quinn, a contemporary of Samuel Hahneman, retailers of homeopathic remedies soon followed. By 1830 Dr James Epps was supplying homeopathic medicine chests. These are much less varied than the orthodox chests, and

CRELLIN'S MAJOR THERAPEUTIC CATEGORIES		OTHER THERAPEUTIC CATEGORIES	
PURGATIVES	eg Tinct. Jalap. Calomel - sometimes present as "Blue Pill" (mercury). Castor Oil. Epsom salts. Glauber salts. Magnesia. Rhubarb. Senna. Tamarinds. Corrosive sublimate - very poisonous, only rarely found.	EMETICS	Ipecacuanha. Tartar emetic (antimony).
		FEVER REMEDIES AND DRUGS TO PROMOTE SWEATING (Diaphoretics)	
			Salt of Wormwood (Potassium carbonate). Dover's powder (Ipecac + opium). Antimony wine. James' Powder (Antimony) - emetic and purgative in large doses. Tinct. Bark (Quinine sulphate from 1820 onwards). "Cooling" drinks such as carbonates and acidic lemon juice were popular, and from the early part of the 19thC. Seidlitz powders appeared (the great success of these contributed to the prosperity of Savory & Moore who held the patent).
STIMULANTS	for "lowness of spirits" or digestive upsets. eg Hartshorn drops. Camphor. Ether. Cayenne pepper. Sal volatile.		
PREPARATIONS FOR EXTERNAL APPLICATION		ANODYNES	Laudanum. Tinct. Opium. Elixir Paregoric English, or Scottish which had twice as much opium, a very popular cough remedy especially for children.
	Opaldeldoc (soap liniment and opium) a very popular remedy for sprains and bruises. Goulard's extract (lead acetate) for burns. Traumatic Balsam or Turlington's Balsam for minor wounds. Various ointments - Blistering. Spermaceti. Yellow Basilicon. Red Precipitate powder (a mercury preparation) for proud flesh.		
		ANTI-CONVULSANTS	
			Tincture of soot.
		ANTI-DIARRHOEAL REMEDIES	
			Chalk mixture. Laudanum.

have rising lids and one or two drawers in the base. Lying horizontally in the drawer are bottles, with ground glass stoppers, of liquids for external application. Wallets of Calendula and Arnica plasters are frequently housed in pockets in the lid lining, and the remaining space is filled with rows and rows of small, round, corked bottles of "pilules" or tinctures. The only apparatus present is a small spoon or a bent glass rod for "dropping the tinctures", these also being accommodated in slots in the lid lining. (Illustration 56).

In great contrast to the orthodox chests, homeopathic versions almost invariably have a book of instruction as an integral part of the chest [20,21].

The results of this system of medicine were impressive. During the cholera epidemic of 1854 for example the mortality rate amongst cholera victims admitted to the London

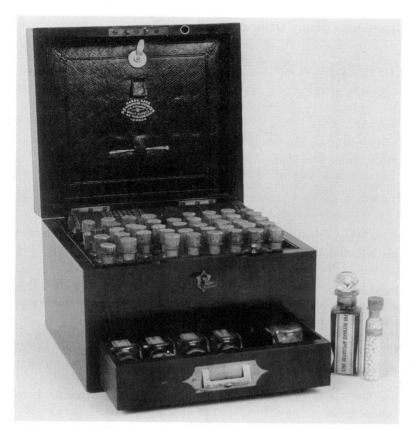

56. Rosewood homeopathic chest by James Epps c1860. 8" x 6". On right, a bottle labelled "FOR OUTWARD APPLICATION ONLY" from drawer, and a bottle of "pilules" from main compartment. A book "Epps Homeopathic Family Instructor" can just be seen at rear of chest

Homeopathic Hospital (founded by Dr Quinn in 1850) was 16.4%, whereas the mortality rate in the other London hospitals was 50%.[22] There are relatively few homeopathic chests in the Wellcome Collection, and this may be because families converted to homeopathy continued to use the remedies until well into the twentieth century.

With the dramatic changes in medicine at the end of the nineteenth century, and the great improvements in communication, the need for cumbersome chests of symptomatic remedies vanished. The "first-aid" needs of travellers and explorers were met by tubes of compressed tablets housed in pocket sized leather wallets or metal cases, and the domestic chests were superseded by the far less elegant bathroom cabinets of modern times.

Some chests, however, live on as treasured antiques or museum exhibits, and one looks back on a few of the old remedies with nostalgia -

> "*Aether*: aether, spirits of Lavender, of each a teaspoonful, mixed with a wine glass full of cold water ... is a good remedy in the hysterical lowness, to which many persons, especially delicate females ... are subject".[23]

NOTES AND REFERENCES

1.   *A Companion to the Medicine Chest with Plain Rules for Taking the Medicines in the Cure of Diseases* by a Member of the Royal College of Surgeons, London. *A New Edition*, 1824. Printed for E Cox & Son. St Thomas Street, Southwark

     Cox's Companion ran to at least 49 editions (or, possibly more correctly, new printings). The 48th - *For Heads of Families, Ship-Captains, Missionaries and Colonists* was published by Simpkin Marshall & Co, London in 1887

2.   Illustration of military chest in *A Prooved Practise for all young Chirurgians*, 1588 by William Clowes

3.   Habrich Christa, Die Ausstattung von Haus - und Reiseapotheken in ihrer Pharmazie und Medizinhistorischen Bedeutung, *Pharmazeutische Zeitung* **124.** Jahrgang Nt 24, 14 Juni 1979

4.   My thanks to Dr Brian Bracegirdle, Keeper, The Wellcome Galleries, Science Museum, London, for kindly allowing me to study these cards, and also to Mr John Burnett of the Science Museum for his unstinted help

5.   Pinto E H, Apothecary Cabinets, *History of Medicine* 1970. **2,** pp 25-27

6.   So called because a handsome chest of this style in the Wellcome Collection reputedly belonged to the Duke of York, younger brother of George III. The Duke of York died in 1763 and a recent study of the chest shows that it was made in 1789 and cannot therefore have belonged to him

7.   Trade card: *Thomas White, Chemist and Druggist, 24 Cornhill, London, 1839,* with illustrations of three medicine chests incorporated in the design

8.   Reece Richard, *A Practical Dictionary of Domestic Medicine*, printed for Longman, Hurst, Rees and Orme, Paternoster Row, London. This includes a plate with engravings of his *Improved Family Dispensary* and his *Country Clergyman's Dispensary*

9.   List of Chemists, and Druggists, labels on medicine chest bottles in the Wellcome Collection. Supplied by courtesy of the Wellcome Institute of the History of Medicine, London

10. Holloway S W F, "The Orthodox Fringe: the origins of the Pharmaceutical Society of Great Britain," *Medical Fringe and Medical Orthodoxy 1750-1850.* Ed W F Bynum and Roy Porter, Croom Helm, 1987, London

11. A tiny one so found: 2" x 3" pp 64. *DIRECTIONS for using THE MEDICINES contained IN THE CHEST.* Prepared by W Brydon & Co 1840, Wholesale Druggists, 29 Abchurch Lane, Lombard Street. Printed by Joseph Rickerby, Sherbourn Lane, London

12. eg: Names of the several medicines, etc, contained in the chest, alphabetically arranged (60 items) and A list of apparatus necessary to be kept in the chest from - Bond J, *A Companion to the Medicine Chest* 3rd Ed c1820. Shaw & Sons, London

13.   eg: "Table of Weights and Measures" from *A Companion to the Medicine Chest* by A Medical Practitioner 13th Ed, 1834. Printed for James Tindal

14.   eg: "Table of Doses proportional to the age of the patient". From the above guide (12). A most confusing table:-

"For an adult ...... 1 Ex 3i

From 21 years to 15 ......3/4 ...... ij, qr.v

down to ....

6 months ...... 1/16 ...... nearly gr. iv

.... 1 month ......1/20 ...... gr. iii"

15.   eg. A list of drugs from Richards H, *Instructions ... The Family Chest*, 1808, London

16.   see: Appendix in *Butler's Medicine Chest Directory*, 3rd Ed, 1832. Printed for Butler's Medical Hall, Dublin. pp 178-179.

17.   Savory J, Member of the Society of Apothecaries, London. *A Companion to the Medicine Chest, or Plain Directions for the Employment of the Various Medicines, etc. Contained in it, with Properties and Doses of such as are more Generally Used in Domestic Medicine*, Churchills, London, 1836

18.   Maw J & S, *A Companion to Maw's New Portable Medicine Chests*, London, c1830

19.   Crellin J K, Domestic Medicine Chests: Microcosms of 18th and 19th century medical practice. *Pharmacy in History*, 1979. **21** No 3, pp 122-131. Also Crellin J K, British Pharmacy and 19th century domestic medicine, *Veroffentichungen - internationalen fur geschichte der Pharmazie* 1969, *32*, pp 81-86

20.   Contained in the Epps chest shown in Illustration 56 - Epps Richard, Surgeon, *The Homeopathic Family Instructor*, c1850, pp 739. Printed for James Epps, London

21.   Another example is a small (3" x 2") black leather covered case inscribed in gold inside the lid of a case by - *W Headland, Homeopathic Chemist, Princes Street, Hanover Square*, containing 24 small glass tubes of "pilules" and also a booklet: *Homeopathic Manual containing Hints for Domestic Practice*, c1860, pp 122

22.   Inglis B, *Natural Medicine*, William Collins & Co, London, 1979, pp48-49

23.   Ibid Ref. 1.

ACKNOWLEDGEMENTS

My thanks to the Antique Collectors' club for giving me permission to use material first published in its journal *"Antique Collecting"*, Dec. 1980 and Jan. 1981 and also to *"Country Life"* for allowing me to use photographs from my article on Domestic Medicine Chests Jan. 31st 1985.

Illustrations: John Young

BATH PHILOSOPHICAL SOCIETY.

THE great Advantages which have been derived from various scientific Institutions in London, Manchester, Liverpool, Newcastle, &c. have induced Dr. WILKINSON to propose the Appropriation of the KINGSTON LECTURE-ROOM to the Purposes of a similar Institution in this City. This Room is already supplied with an extensive Assortment of Philosophical and Chemical Apparatus, Furnaces, &c. calculated for the Illustration of most Subjects connected with the Arts and Manufactures.

It is presumed that all Gentlemen interested in any of the various Objects relative to the different Branches of Experimental Philosophy, Chemistry, Geology, Mineralogy, and their Applications to the Arts, Manufactures, Agriculture, &c. would derive considerable Advantages from being Members of a Society, formed of some who may be acquainted with the Principles of the different Sciences, and of others, who, from being engaged in Commercial and Manufacturing Establishments, are capable of imparting valuable practical Information.

Hence it will be desirable to have among its Members such as, from their Occupations, are engaged in Iron Founderies, Breweries, Glass-Houses, &c. and that all respectable Commercial and Agricultural Persons be deemed admissible to the Institution.

To Parents, it will afford a desirable Opportunity of a weekly rational Recreation to their Sons: by thus early expanding their minds, it may contribute considerably to their future Respectability in Society.

With these objects in View, the following Plan is respectfully submitted to the Public:

1st, That the Meetings of the Society be on every MONDAY Evening during the Year, excepting the Months of July, August, and September, at half-past Seven, and to close at half-past Nine.

2d, The first Hour to be appropriated to the Communication from any of its Members of different interesting Subjects connected with the Objects of the Society, and of Proposals relative to Experiments desired to be tried. The second Hour, to the Reading and Discussion of any Paper presented to the Society, or to any Lecture volunteered by any of its Members.

In Case there should be no Subject Matter for Discussion before the Society, then Dr. W. engages to deliver an Experimental Lecture on some Branch of Natural Philosophy or Chemistry.

3d, That each Member shall be intitled to introduce each Evening a Lady, or a Young Gentleman under 16 Years of Age.

4th, That all Members of this Society shall be free to all the Lectures delivered by Dr. WILKINSON, in the Kingston Lecture-Room.

5th, After the first Meeting of the Society, each Person subsequently admitted as a Member, must be reccommended by two Subscribers to the Institution.

6th, That there will be three Presidents, a Secretary, and an Experimentalist.

7th, Each Subscriber to pay, on his Admission, Two Guineas and Five Shillings, and the same paid annually.

8th, Visitors to Bath may be admitted as Members for Three Months, upon being properly introduced, and upon paying One Guinea and Five Shillings.

The First Meeting to take place on MONDAY, Dec. 11th.

☞ *Gentlemen disposed to become Members, are requested to have their Names entered in the Society's Subscription-Book at the Kingston Pump-Room.*

WOOD and Co. *Printers of the Bath and Cheltenham Gazette,* 9, UNION-STREET, BATH.

57. Proposals for the third Bath Philosophical Society.

THE FOUR BATH PHILOSOPHICAL SOCIETIES 1779-1959

Hugh Torrens

It is remarkable, in a city like Bath whose history has so *often* been examined, that the histories of science and of technology have received so little attention; a notable exception being the book by Williams and Stoddart.[1] Such lacunae seem all the more strange when we consider that two significant scientists of the eighteenth and early nineteenth centuries, namely William Herschel (1738-1822), the astronomer and William Smith (1769-1839), the geologist, both made their major advances in the Bath area. But the intellectual, economic and technological characteristics of the Bath world in which these developments took place, have been very little studied. The welcome work of Neale[2] has done nothing to correct this bias.

By 1800 the popularity of Bath as a resort was unchallenged. There was an extraordinary number of transport services to and from London, to bring the visitors (of whom 5,281 were individually listed in that year's *Bath Journal*) and, after 1800, progressively larger numbers of residents, back and forth to Bath. To service the same people a total of 62 physicians, surgeons, druggists, and chemists are listed in the 1790's.[3] But how did such visitors and residents pass the often large amounts of their leisure time in Bath? Did the traditional search for pleasure or marriage partners pictured so well by many (like Whiston)[4] apply to all? What was serious intellectual life like in the Bath of this period? Barbeau,[5] in what has proved an unfortunately influential book, claimed that in eighteenth century Bath there "was little desire for literary or scientific knowledge". This paper tries to show that such a judgment is seriously premature, by documenting something of the activities of the several Philosophical Societies based there.

The Philosophical Society movement in England has been characterised by many historians as closely connected with the rise of industrialisation,[6] while the Manchester Literary and Philosophical Society, founded in 1781 in this industrial centre, is consistently and misleadingly recorded as the oldest provincial learned Society in England,[7,8,9,] Porter[10] has provided a stimulating corrective view. The existence of the earliest known Philosophical Society in Bath is most clearly recorded on the title pages of books produced by members, like Edmund Rack (1735-1787) and Matthew Martin (1748-1838). Such volumes were published at least between 1781 (the title page recording Rack's secretaryship of "the Philosophical Society lately instituted at Bath")[11] and 1786,[12] proving that there was a Philosophical Society in Bath over this period, although nothing is recorded for Bath in McClellan's survey.[13]

In relation to the essentially unimportant questions of precise priority, and the more interesting connections such Societies had to the processes of industrialisation, the situation is clearly more complex than has been realised. Bath, so often regarded as a city indifferent, even hostile, to industry, and one proudly and misleadingly proclaimed, even as late as 1855, as "not a City of trade ... with no manufacture worthy of notice carried on within its limits, ... and not the resort of commerce",[14] emerges as a city highly active in the formation, if not in the maintenance, of such Societies.

The first relevant Society in Bath was the "Society for the encouragement of Agriculture, Arts, Manufactures and Commerce", founded in 1777, and which came to involve itself more and more with agriculture. This Society survives to this day, as the Bath and West of England Agricultural Society.[15] Not long afterwards, a different and more "Select Society" was instituted, on 28th December 1779, as the first Bath Philosophical Society. The printed rules of this survive in the library of the Royal Society (Blagden archives).

The early months of this Society and its evolution are well documented in the MSS journal of the first Secretary of both these Societies, Edmund Rack, now preserved in Bath Reference Library. From this, and the original manuscripts of the 32 papers which William Herschel read to the Society between January 1780 and March 1781, we get a good idea of the range of activities which the Society fostered. The rules record that "any subject within the circle of the Arts and Sciences, Natural History, the History of Nations, or any branch of Polite Literature" was judged acceptable, as were "essays on Morality, and the Social Virtues, with candid criticisms of new poetical, scientific and philosophical publications and new Translations from Foreign Authors", but "for obvious reasons, Law, Physic, Divinity and Politics" were to be wholly excluded from debate at the Society.

Herschel's papers discussed physical and astronomical topics in the main, with philosophy and metaphysics. Only one contribution, which was significantly also Herschel's first, was in the field of natural history. It would be wrong to regard this as of little interest to the Society's membership. In fact the Society was active across the whole of natural history,[16] which was one of significance for Herschel too.[17] One writer has suggested that the main focus of the Society was specifically geological,[18] but this is a distortion drawing on the only aspect of the Society's activities which has been documented.

To the first Society's 27 members[19] a few more can now be added, to bring the total to 31. These are Dr Matthew Dobson (1727-1784)[20] and Dr James Johnstone[21] with two further Honorary members, Dr John Grieve (1742-1805)[22] and Dr Richard Pulteney (1730-1801).[23] When we consider that only four of these 31 are listed as Honorary Members (the other two in this category are Drs Charles Blagden and John Coakley Lettsom), and that the rules specified there were to be no more than twenty five ordinary members when the Society was founded in 1779, it seems likely that the membership of this Society now on record is an accurate reflection of its actual membership.

The Society intended to publish its *Transactions* but never did. Those original extracts from the Secretary's transcript of the papers read, which were in the Herschel archive and are now at Harvard University, show that the original Minutes were later dispersed among the members.

The Society also intended to build up a library, but, if it did, no books from it are known to have survived. It met in a room at the circulating library run by Martha Bally at 11 Milsom Street in Bath. Of the 31 members, 15 (48%) appear in the *Dictionary of National Biography (hereafter D.N.B.)*, the same proportion, but not the same members, were

Fellows of the Royal Society (F.R.S.), whatever that honour meant during Sir Joseph Banks' presidency.[24] The contribution of the 12 (40%) medical men (which includes two surgeons) is also remarkable. Of the ten with M D degrees, that eight were trained in part or wholly at Edinburgh, suggests that Schnorrenberg's assessment[25] that "the tide of Scots trained physicians did not (then) seem particularly noticeable in Bath" needs correction.

Of the activities of the Society, apart from meetings, we have little record. But two members are known to have undertaken industrial espionage of the "new technology" of Jonathan Hornblower's compound steam engine in 1782, soon after it was erected at Radstock near Bath, in 1781.[26] This spying was undertaken by members James Collings and Dr William Watson, on behalf of Matthew Boulton and James Watt, the steam engineering partnership based in Birmingham. Collings had been an active member of the "Club of Honest Whigs" in London and had attended a Lunar Society meeting at Birmingham before he settled in Bath, and Watson, with two other members of the Bath Society, was soon to sponsor Watt's election to the Royal Society in 1785. The potential for such co-operation between the members of the many scientific and philosophical Societies in eighteenth century England was clearly enormous, even if it is now so difficult to chronicle.

In eighteenth century Bath the make-up of leisured and educated society changed from year to year, as people came and went. This is well reflected by the first Bath Society. First Joseph Priestley left for Birmingham in 1780 when death also claimed its first member, then Herschel left for London in 1781. The founder of the Society, Thomas Curtis, died in 1784, the same year another member, Dr John Staker, took his own life. In 1787 the Secretary Edmund Rack died, and with him the first Bath Philosophical Society came to a natural, and typically Bathonian, end. The Philosophical Society's very success in promoting the provincial Herschel to a metropolitan status also made any momentum the Society had developed that much harder to sustain.

But the appetite for such a body clearly continued, however fitfully. A second Bath Philosophical Society was founded ten years later on 11th December 1798. We know this, and that at least Watson and Herschel of the first Society, were elected members, from the record by Frederick Shum (1822-1916) from the first MSS minute book of this Society and covering the period 1798 to 1801. This volume was still extant in 1913,[27] but all attempts to trace it since have failed.[28] Despite its loss, thirteen members of this Society have been identified and the Society's survival until at least 1805 can be documented. Of these thirteen, four were members of the first Society, ten (77%) are listed in *D.N.B.*, eight (62%) were F.R.S. and eight (62%), but not the same eight, were medical men including John Haygarth (1740-1827).

William Smith's geological discoveries were certainly being circulated, before they had been properly published, in the period 1799-1815.[29] There has been debate about the extent to which (if at all) this happened. A recent writer has claimed that Smith had "few contacts with the leisured amateurs who (then) made up the bulk of the English geological community".[30] However this second Bath Philosophical Society was active just when Smith was still based in Bath, before his migration to London in 1803. The fact that 40% of the documented members of the second Bath Society are known associates of Smith, suggests that this Society, then based in the most popular resort in Britain, could have been as significant in advancing Smith's career, as the first Society was in advancing Herschel's. When we realise that the Bath and West of England Agricultural Society also established a Chemical Laboratory there in 1807, at which Smith's stratigraphic methods were further disseminated, we may suspect that Smith's connection with Bath was especially fortunate, for someone who took longer to publish than has been good for his reputation among some historians of science.

The third Bath Philosophical Society was the brainchild of one man, a remarkable medic, called Charles Hunnings Wilkinson (1763/4-1850).[31] He had settled in Bath by 1806, and by 1808 had also acquired (or perhaps awarded himself!) an MD degree. Here he established himself as a medical and scientific lecturer and became the proprietor of the Kingston Hot Bath, where he had built a Lecture Room by 1811. Here he lectured on Experimental Philosophy, Chemistry and Mineralogy, as he records in a volume published in 1811 on the Bath Waters.[32] Wilkinson's lectures once again drew attention to the importance of Smith's results and further helped to disseminate them, through the stratigraphically-arranged collection of fossils, which Wilkinson placed on display in his lecture room.

Wilkinson is a fascinating larger-than-life character, of whom Peach[33] recorded; "the doctor *went into* everything; nothing was above or beneath his grasp; it was amazing to hear him theorise upon every new invention and dogmatise upon every conceivable topic". In December 1815 Wilkinson issued *Proposals* for a third Bath Philosophical Society. It is obvious from this that it was, in a very real sense, a semi-commercial operation by Wilkinson, who hoped that such a Society would attract patrons to his lectures, including ladies and young gentlemen under sixteen, who would pay a subscription fee for the privilege. Records of this Society are very elusive, but nine members including one woman, have been identified, and the Society is known to have continued until about 1821. It (or rather Wilkinson) certainly survived the Seditious Meetings Act of 1817.[34]

But once again, either the momentum could not be maintained or the social stratification which so easily developed in a place like Bath started to intrude on the Philosophical scene. In the 1820's the cultural and intellectual life of Bath seems to have separated and diversified along class and occupational lines. The upper levels of the country and town gentry, and the higher professionals gathered behind a fourth Bath Society, which was called The Literary and Scientific Institution of Bath. The lower levels of artisans, tradesmen and the lower professionals, with Wilkinson, put their energies into the Bath Mechanics Institute which opened in 1825.[35,36] The former, which had been suggested in 1819, had opened the year before in 1824. Similar tensions between "gentlemanly" science and its more applied aspirations emerge from the recent study of the formation of the Yorkshire Geological and Polytechnic Society in the next decade.[37]

This last, and longest surviving, Bath "Philosophical Society" has had its historians[38] and it published *Reports*, at first annually, but as time went on more irregularly, which allow its proceedings, and the treasures it accumulated, to be investigated in greater detail than for any of the other Societies.[39] The priority of this new organisation, which was graced with Royal patronage from 1830, was the need for a permanent home, where a Museum could be fostered and a Library built up. This opened in January 1825, in Terrace Walk; when the inaugural address was given by that pillar of local scientific society, Sir George Smith Gibbes (1771-1851) F.R.S. 1796, M D 1799.[40] Gibbes had earlier been a member of the second Bath Society and was then an acknowledged part of the Bath scientific scene. He should not be labelled, as he has been by Schnorrenberg[41] "a more alarming kind of quack", a judgement clouded by the prolific satirical literature of Bath. The fact that premises were at last available gave a focus for members' activities which all earlier Societies had lacked. The donation books and annual reports (many of which survive as a valuable Victorian archive) show how much the study of geology and other sciences was encouraged. In 1853 the Museum was greatly extended by the addition of the major geological collections of Charles Moore (1815-1881), to which he made additions up to his death.

But the very nature of Bath society again militated against any long lasting success for the Institution. Charles Henry Parry wrote in 1829, only five years after its formation, that the Institution was then "chiefly sought as a place for Newspapers and Pamphlets & Easy Chairs and heated Air. In addition to this misfortune, that Bath itself cannot support such an Establishment, this has the ill-luck to be placed where no one can reach it".[42] By 1895 a visitor to the Museum of the Institution could write of his "feeling deep and just indignation ...(its state was) a disgrace to any body of educated men at the end of the nineteenth century".[43] The collections, libraries and/or archives of men of the calibre of Moore, Leonard Jenyns (1800-1893) and Christopher Broome (1812-1886) have survived all this, but to an unknown degree, and their transfer to Local Authority control in 1959. The legacy of such cumulative neglect continues in a very real sense today.[44,45] The collections urgently need cataloguing and a permanent, properly maintained, home.

The legacy of this 200 years of scientific and "philosophical" activity in Bath is impossible to quantify. But it is vital to take it into account when assessing the emergence of the two great scientists, with which we started this paper. Above all, more detailed research into such aspects of the history of Bath is needed.[46] For far too long, people have accepted the highly distorted view that has come down, that there was simply no significant scientific or industrial activity in "polite" Bath. This is a view which cannot now be credibly sustained.

REFERENCES

1.   Williams W J and Stoddart D M, *Bath: Some encounters with Science*. Bath: Kingsmead, 1978

2.   Neale R S, *Bath 1680-1850: A Social History*. London: Routledge & Kegan Paul, 1981

3.   McIntyre S, *Towns as health and pleasure resort: Bath, Scarborough and Weymouth 1700-1815*. D.Phil thesis: Oxford University, 1973

4.   Whiston B, *Rare Doings at Bath*. Chicago: Art Institute, 1978

5.   Barbeau A, *Life and Letters at Bath in the XVIIIth Century.* London: Heinemann, 1904

6.   Musson A E and Robinson E, *Science and Technology in the Industrial Revolution.* Manchester: University Press, 1969

7.   Eliot W, Opening Address. *Transactions of the Botanical Society of Edinburgh,* 1871, **11**, pp 11-33

8.   McKie D, Scientific Societies to the end of the Eighteenth Century, in A Ferguson (editor). *Natural Philosophy through the Eighteenth Century and Allied Topics.* pp 133-34, London: Taylor and Francis, 1948

9.   Edmonds J M, The Geological Lecture-Courses given in Yorkshire by William Smith and John Phillips 1824-1825. *Proceedings of the Yorkshire Geological Society,* 1975, **40**, pp 373-412

10. Porter R, Science, Provincial Culture and Public Opinion in Enlightenment England. *British Journal for Eighteenth Century Studies,* 1980, 1980, **3**, pp 20-46

11. Rack E, *Essays, Letters and Poems.* Bath: Cruttwell, 1781

12. Martin M, *Observations on Marine Vermes, Insects, etc.* Exeter: Trewman, 1786, (for the author)

13. Mc Clellan J E III, *Science Reorganised. Scientific Societies in the Eighteenth Century.* New York: Columbia University Press, 1985

14. Gibbs S, *Gibbs's Illustrated Bath Visitant or New Guide to Bath.* Bath; (1855)

15. Hudson K, *The Bath and West: a Bicentenary History.* Bradford on Avon: Moonraker Press, 1976

16. Torrens H S, Geological Communication in the Bath area in the last half of the Eighteenth Century, in L J Jordanova and R Porter (editors). *Images of the Earth*, British Society for the History of Science, Monograph no. 1, Chalfont St Giles, 1976, pp 215-247

17. Schaffer S, Herschel in Bedlam: Natural History and Stellar Astronomy. *British Journal for the History of Science*, 1980, **13**, pp 211-39

18. Russell C, *Science and Social Change 1700-1900.* London: Macmillan, 1983

19. Turner A J, *Science and Music in Eighteenth Century Bath.* Bath: University, 1977

20. Torrens H S, Geological Communication in the Bath area in the last half of the Eighteenth Century, in L J Jordanova and R Porter (editors). *Images of the Earth*, British Society for the History of Science, Monograph no. 1, Chalfont St Giles 1979, pp 215-247

21. Johnstone C L, *History of the Johnstones 1191-1909.* Edinburgh and London: W & A K Johnston Ltd, 1909

22. Appleby J H, John Grieve's Correspondence with Joseph Black and Some Contemporaneous Russo-Scottish Medical Intercommunication. *Medical History*, 1985, **29**, pp 401-13

23. Jeffers R H, Richard Pulteney M D, F R S (1730-1801) and his correspondents. *Proceedings of the Linnean Society*, 1960, **171**, pp 15-26

24. Anon, A Review of some leading points in the Official Character and Proceedings of the late President of the Royal Society. *Philosophical Magazine*, 1820, **56**, pp 161-74, 241-57

25. Schnorrenberg B B, Medical Men of Bath. *Studies in Eighteenth Century Culture*, 1984, **13**, pp 189-203

26. Torrens H S, Winwoods of Bristol: part one 1767-1788. *Bristol Industrial Archaeology Society Journal*, 1980, **13**, pp 9-17

27. Shum F, *A Catalogue of Bath Books ... collected by F Shum*. Bath: Simms, 1913

28. Torrens H S, Bath Philosophical Societies. *Notes and Queries*, 1986, **231**, p 195

29. Torrens H S, Hawking History - A Vital Future for Geology's Past. *Modern Geology,* 1988, **12**, pp 1-11

30. Laudan R, *From Mineralogy to Geology: The Foundations of a Science 1650-1850*. University of Chicago Press 1987, p 158

31. Thornton J L, Charles Hunnings Wilkinson (1763 or 64 - 1850). *Annals of Science*, 1967, **23**, pp 277-86

32. Wilkinson C H, *Analytical Researches into the Properties of the Bath Waters (etc)*. Bath: Wood and Cunningham, 1811

33. Peach R E, *Historic Houses in Bath and their associations*. London: Simpkin, Marshall and Co. and Bath: Peach, 1883

34. Inkster I, Seditious Science: a reply to Paul Weindling. *British Journal for the History of Science*, 1981, **14**, pp 181-8

35. Neale R S, *Economic Conditions and Working Class Movements in the City of Bath 1800-50*. M A thesis: Bristol University 1962

36. Williams W J and Stoddart D M, *Bath: Some encounters with Science*. Bath: Kingsmead 1978

37. Morrell J. The early Yorkshire Geological and Polytechnic Society: a reconsideration. *Annals of Science*, **45**, pp 153-67, 1988

38. Hunter J, *The Connection of Bath with the Literature and Science of England*. Bath: Cruttwell 1827. Reprinted with additional material. Bath: Peach and London: Parker 1853

39.   Copp C et al The Bath Geological Collections. *Newsletter of the Geological Curators Group*, 1975, **1**, (3), pp 88-124

40.   Gibbes G S, *Address delivered at the opening of the Bath Literary and Philosophical Institution*. Bath, 1825: Higman (printer)

41.   Schnorrenberg B B, Medical Men of Bath. *Studies in Eighteenth Century Culture*, 1984, **13**, pp 189-203

42.   Parry C H, MSS letter to William Salmond, dated July 24, 1829. Bodleian library, Oxford: MSS Engl. Misc. d 612, p 140

43.   Anon, The Bath Literary and Philosophical Institution. *Natural Science*, 1895, **7**, pp 370-1

44.   Greenslade B et al. *Letter to the Charity Commissioners on the Bath Royal Literary and Scientific Institution* dated 5 August, 1987. (Copy in Bath Geological Museum).

45.   Profit J, Battle looms on dusty treasures. *Bath and West of England Evening Chronicle*, April 29, 1988, p 9

46.   Porter R, Science, Provincial Culture and Public Opinion in Enlightenment England. *British Journal for Eighteenth Century Studies*, 1980, **3**, pp 20-46

THE CHANGING PUBLIC ESTIMATE OF THE MEDICAL PROFESSION IN NINETEENTH CENTURY BRISTOL

Patricia Maureen Craig

The British Medical Association held three annual general meetings in Bristol during the nineteenth century. The first of these meetings, in 1833,[1] was very briefly and formally announced in the several weekly papers published in Bristol at the time.[2] The meetings of 1863 and especially that of 1894 were much more extensively reported, particularly in the *Western Daily Press*. This essay compares the coverage of the two meetings in that paper.

The purpose of the comparison is to attempt to answer the question asked by John Addington Symonds in his presidential address to the Annual General Meeting of the BMA in 1863:

> "How has the art of medicine advanced in the opinion of the public, since the last meeting of the BMA in the city in 1833?"

They met there again in 1894. How might the changing public view of the profession during those sixty years be gauged? Symonds looked to the press for an opinion and we shall see later what he found.

On the day they gathered for their meeting in 1863, the medical profession found itself under attack from the editor of the local paper:[3]

> "It is astonishing to what extent society suffers itself to be quacked, medically speaking."

He continued with a version of Montaigne's fable, the one describing how a physician actually brings illness to a village where it had not been experienced before and how the arrival of a second physician actually increases the variety of illnesses. "Two lawyers may live in a town, but one cannot."

From this very critical start the tone of the leading article changes, though retaining a note of scepticism.

> "The truly qualified English Medical Practitioner is, in 99 cases out of 100, a man of rare worth in society but in large mining and manufacturing districts there is still a class of medical practitioners who merit all the suspicion which the popular mind with its usual lack of discrimination has attached to the profession generally."

There follows a passage in a different tone:

> "Our medical men, with few exceptions are men who have given their lives to their work. By long and patient preliminary study of the anatomy and functions of the human frame, the varied forms of disease that attack vitality more or less directly, the nature of medicines and their operation both in the sick and the healthy, they

have prepared themselves at universities and hospitals for being admitted members of the healing guild. Though they will encounter later things they did not see in their training, it has stood them in good stead. They must advise on the laws of health and tell people to consult them and to avoid quacks. Though doctors practice an uncertain art, long training makes them better."

The article ends with a compliment:

"None of the learned professions is so liberal in unpaid labours as the healing profession."

This article was published on the 5th August, the day upon which Symonds[4] delivered his presidential address. A *verbatim* report of this of one column's length appeared on August 6th. Like the previous day's leading article this address, given just five years after the passage of the Medical Registration Act, starts on a note of scepticism, not the speaker's but that of quoted sources, and ends with a plea for medical training to be seen as a justification for confidence in the medical profession. Symonds quoted the *Saturday Review* of 11th October 1862 which had said "medicine (is) not an approved science"; the *London Review* of 24th January 1863 "charged the profession with empiricism". After elaborating the points about the value of medical training which had been made in the previous day's leader Symonds urged the dubious to see for themselves "the medical schools, dissecting rooms, laboratories and private studios" when they would surely be convinced that medicine is a science, though it would always be an art also, because each patient had to be treated as a unique individual.

On the 7th and 8th of August the paper carried reports of scientific papers read at the meeting. The four major addresses were given by well-known local doctors so it is of interest to see that two were reported at length and two only very briefly. Augustin Prichard's[5] talk on carbuncles was briefly dismissed; somewhat boring? That of Joseph Swayne[6] on the use of chloroform was similarly given short shrift. Did this reflect a low estimate of women, or obstetricians, or was the subject thought indelicate? Certainly the paper given by William Budd[7] seems in retrospect a seminal contribution to the understanding of epidemiology. It was given coverage of one column, as was the paper by William Bird Herapath, on chemistry. Budd gave an account of an outbreak of sheep pox in Wiltshire in which he set out the reasons why investigating a limited epidemic in which all variables could be controlled was of much greater value than using the method, popular with the BMA at the time, of collecting vast amounts of information about the circumstances, most of which were irrelevant. Budd was able to support the conclusion that this was a disease specific to sheep, contagious, and passed on by a virus[8] which multiplied in the victim's body.

In contrast to Budd's very clear account of his work Herapath, reported on 8th August, gave a review of the whole of chemistry to that date which is just overwhelming and confusing. However, the following passage stands out:

"Chemistry as loudly protests against the Mosaic record being true in a strictly liberal sense as does geology, geography or any other of the physical sciences, so absurdly dogmatised upon weekly from the pulpits."

This was just four years after the publication of *The Origin of Species* and did provoke a protest at the meeting, but there was neither editorial comment nor angry letters to the paper about it, even though the next week the paper published a further extract. This was done by request, though we are not told whose. The additional paragraphs reinforce a Deist message.

Dr Herapath was also one of the stars of the first event of the social programme which took place in the Literary and Philosophical Institute in Park Street on the evening of the 6th August. This was a scientific affair at which various local people demonstrated work, Herapath having on display a microscope for which he won a gold medal in Paris in 1851, Mr Philips of Weston super Mare demonstrated electric light. He did so again at the soiree held at the home of A.J. Symonds the following evening.[9] On the final night of the conference there was a dinner attended by the Mayor and Mr Commissioner Hill, in the Victoria Rooms, the main venue for the meeting. "The gallery was well occupied by a very large number of ladies."

In 1894 the meeting was longer and larger in every way. It may be only because of that, that it received six to seven times as much coverage as the 1863 meeting. However, the tone of the coverage, as well as the content of the meeting, was quite different.

First a brief look at two kinds of coverage that were not given in 1863: related features and related advertising. On the opening day the Congress - (the paper's word for this meeting) there was a full page feature describing all Bristol's medical associations. There are brief histories and descriptions of eleven Bristol medical institutions[10] and biographies of a number of distinguished physicians who had worked in Bristol include those of A.J. Symonds and William Budd. A feature describing the beauties of the city and its surroundings ends:

> "When physicians who are visiting us find their patients anxious to know where to settle down, they will know what a place to recommend."

On the second and third days of the congress, full page advertisements for Vinolia Soap, directed to the medical profession, appeared in the paper.

There were leading articles, sometimes two, every day from 31st July to the 4th August. As with the leader at the beginning of the meeting in 1863 that upon 31st July echoes, or rather prefigures, the president's opening address. The others take a particular speech from the previous day's meeting which is elsewhere quoted at length, and present a summary. There is no expression of editorial opinion; the medical views are presented as authoritative. But of course there was selection for comment of a small amount from much material.

How was the choice determined? A first consideration was obviously local interest. The President, Edward Long Fox, and Bristol's Professor of Surgery, James Greig Smith[11] were the only major speakers from the city. The other speakers singled out were dealing with a particular range of issues, bacteriology, public health, the regulatory function of the medical profession in this field and another area, that of mental health, including alcohol abuse, where the profession could be perceived to have a role in controlling deviance and supporting the state in the maintenance of order.

Greig Smith's paper fell somewhat outside this field being concerned with the training of surgeons in their craft. He is at pains to point out that he thinks standards of surgery in Britain very good and is suggesting improvements, not radical change. That sums up the ethos of this meeting.

On the 1st of August a second leader informs us that many participants had come from the Public Health Congress. What stamina they had! At that meeting Cardinal Vaughan had commented favourably upon the provision in Germany, of winter gardens for workers. This brings out three themes to which both comment in the leaders and quotations from speeches at the congress keep returning. First there are a number of allusions to things being done better in Germany. Long Fox asks:

> "Is it not remarkable that in a practical country (Britain) the existence of institutions for medical education and research depends upon private charity"[12] unlike the continent, especially Germany?

Sir Charles Alexander Cameron, speaking on public health pointed out that in this country there were no medically qualified privy councillors, (unlike Germany!). But, he went on to say that, the "upheaval of the lower strata to the upper crust", then said to be taking place, might bring members of the profession to a better level in the corridors of power.[13] Secondly, there was much stress laid upon encouraging the workers to be sober responsible family men. But thirdly, and here the paper showed its Tory colour, there was caution about spending public money. However, when Sir Charles demanded "increased centralised control" the editor described this as "not an unmixed blessing but necessary in matters of health".

There was a very special local concern about sewers. Whilst elsewhere the argument was not whether but by what means sewers should be ventilated, Bristol's own sewers were unventilated. The paper was pleased to support the City's Medical Officer of Health, Dr D.S. Davies when he pointed out that, despite this, Bristol's health record compared favourably with that of most large cities. The expense of installing a new sewage system would have been a heavy burden on the *Western Daily Press*'s rate paying readers.

The opening of the Clifton Pump Room and Spa by George Newnes, MP was an important local event which had been timed, so that, as a leader on the subject put it, it could "take place in medical week".

The leading articles are so bland that it must be esteemed a compliment to the female sex that in welcoming the BMA to the city on 31st July we learn that "incidentally it is *worthwhile* to note that this is the first congress to which ladies holding medical qualification will be admitted".[14] They get no further mention. Any sort of comment on personalities or interview with individuals is entirely absent, nor did the public comment by way of letters. "The profession is now established and accepted. The BMA is welcome. Its growth is a safeguard of the public interest".[14] The items to be discussed during the forthcoming meeting which are singled out for comment, underline the profession's role as an instrument of social control, sometimes in most unexceptionable ways, sometimes questionably authoritarian. The Pharmacy Act, seeking to prevent the inclusion of poisons in proprietary medicines or the Railway Act including a requirement to see that those needing to interpret signals were not colour blind, could only be welcomed. However, the compulsory therapeutic seclusion of drunkards could be abused, as could the assessment of the mental condition of school children. The editor makes no such judgement, simply accepting all these suggestions with no warning of the need for caution. There is a welcome too for a discussion of the means to prevent "abuse" of charity.

On the 1st August, under the heading *The Medical Man and the State*, the paper comments upon Edward Long Fox's presidential speech of which a large extract is given on another page. As they say he "descanted upon the relations of the medical man and the State". This passage deals characteristically with his most important themes.

> "What are the advantages of our numbers? What the benefits of our knowledge of the wants of mankind, and of the modes of their relief, if we are not, from time to time to assert our claims to be, even more than we are at present, the advisers of the State. As a profession we are above party. Our highest aspirations tend to the formation of a pure commonwealth. The poor, the sick, the criminal are our daily study, primarily for the relief of the individual, but with nobler and far reaching aims namely that poverty may be mitigated by more healthy surroundings, that sickness may be diminished by the education of the nation in the wiser laws of health, by increased temperance and by knowledge from an early age of the common facts of physiology, and that the criminal class in the future may occupy narrower limits because they are no longer the victims of a debased they are heredity. Poverty disease and crime are the objects of our investigations as a profession; these are the foul blots in the State for which we seek amelioration."

Fox points out, as mentioned earlier, that the German state does better by medicine than the British and that all Jenner got was the gratitude of patients. And now the "crazy cry of liberty of the subject" is limiting the effectiveness of vaccination. Though paternalistic, Fox appears most humane and in this passage is asking for something we still seem unable to provide properly today. "Homes for them" (the mad and feebleminded), "what is the good of sending these poor creatures to prison over and over again? They need homes, not asylums or penal settlements."

Editorially, the paper picks up Fox's views but gives them a harsher emphasis.

There is not space to give a detailed account of the social programme. Set out in tabular form, it is seen to be very crowded. It is different in character too from that of 1863, giving much more of interest to what the BMA today describes as "accompanying persons".

Emphasis of a few points tells us more about the profession's view of itself and the public view of the profession than all the verbiage in the leaders. Temperance was an important issue, the subject of the only things recognisable as "fringe meetings". Lewis Fry was a great benefactor and fund raiser for the University College. Clearly he and the Merchant Venturers who were supporting the rival Technical College wanted to gain the support of the profession. So too, as potential educators of their offspring, did Clifton College and the Bristol Grammar School. The exhibition at the Drill Hall all week was arguably more scientific than social, so too perhaps the visit to the waterworks. Otherwise only brief glimpses of the Mineral Water Hospital at Bath, and Jenner's old home at Berkeley remind us this was a medical gathering. It is a *social* programme with ladies in mind.

At the closing function 1,800 ladies and gentlemen attended including all the civic dignitaries, two MPs, the High Sheriff and so on, or as the paper says: "The most imposing gathering which has been seen in Bristol for years".[15] There was dancing, and supper was served from 11 pm to batches of 500.

And if you think they were all worn out they were not. Many were up with the lark for Saturday excursions in great style, by special train or steamer or huge horse drawn conveyances. At Berkeley, Lord Fitzharding personally helped to show them round. The profession seems to have felt at this time it was not appropriately recognised by the national London establishment but it was certainly thought very important in a provincial city.

How does that compare with the situation in 1863 as measured by the coverage in the *Western Daily Press*?

If we include a possibly related article on sewers in the week following the meeting, the coverage in 1863 was about ten columns. The total in 1894, when the paper still had the same total of eight pages, was about sixty-five columns. Why was this?

First, the 1894 meeting was much longer, five days including Saturday excursion, against three in 1863. Also in 1894 many different events both scientific and social were going on at the same time. It is not possible to prove that this in itself was not the whole explanation of the longer coverage.

Second, it appears from the nature of the coverage, for example printing the day's programmes in advance, that the paper was directing its coverage as much to the participants in the meeting as to the general reading public.

Third, the whole tone of the coverage is quite different, almost sycophantic in its praise for the profession. It seems reasonable to think that the paper's increased coverage of the meeting reflects a different view of the authority and importance of the profession, perhaps particularly in the provinces, than that which prevailed in 1863.

The BMA had about 15,000 members in 1894 but only 2,200 in 1863. It was a much larger and more important group in the later year with a high opinion of its own achievements. At the very least the editorial line of the *Western Daily Press* does not question this view.

In 1863 medicine could be described, to use Kuhn's[16] terms, as undergoing a change of paradigm. It was a fairly early stage of the development of the germ theory and Budd, certainly, could be described as doing revolutionary science. In selecting Budd's paper and that of Herapath, with its allusions to the debates about the origins of the world and our species, for long reports, the *Western Daily Press* was recognising, albeit without wholly understanding the phenomenon, the importance of these papers in the development of new thinking.

By 1894 medicine, particularly in relation to infectious disease had entered a phase of normal science. This very necessary period of consolidation gave rise to a meeting in which the content was worthy but not exciting. The excitement then lay more in the social activities engaged in by a profession newly established.

SOCIAL PROGRAMME FOR THE 1863 AND 1894 MEETING

1863		
WEDNESDAY 5th AUGUST	THURSDAY 8th AUGUST	FRIDAY 7th AUGUST
Conversazione at Literary & Philosophical Institute	Soiree at Clifton Hill House	Dinner at Victoria Rooms

1894				
TUESDAY 31st JULY	WEDNESDAY 1st AUGUST	THURSDAY 2nd AUGUST	FRIDAY 3rd AUGUST	SATURDAY 4th AUGUST
Service at 3pm Cathedral	AM Opening of Clifton Spa and Pump Room Garden Party given by Lewis Fry at Goldney House Conversazione at Clifton College Concert at The Zoo Temperance Meeting YMCA	Temperance Breakfast Excursion to the docks 11.00am Garden Party Ashton Court 2-4pm Bristol Grammar School 3-5pm Smoking Concert Banquet	Excursion to Bath with lunch and reception Luncheon with Merchant Venturers Visits Clevedon Bristol Waterworks Reception Colston Hall	All Day Excursions 1. Lynmouth and Ilfracombe 2. Weston super Mare and Cheddar 3. Tortworth and Berkeley 4. Wells and Glastonbury 5. Tintern

Coverage of BMA AGM's in the Western Daily Press	1863	1894
Leading Articles	1·5	7
	+ (2)	
Presidents Address	1	3
Other Keynote Speeches	2·5	6
Scientific Papers	0·5	6
Social Programme	2·5	17
Associated Features	0	12
Associated Advertising	0	16
TOTAL (COLUMNS)	10	67
SIZE OF PAPER (PAGES)	8	8
NUMBER OF DAYS OF MEETING	4	6

NOTES & REFERENCES

1.   P. Craig, "The First BMA meeting in Bristol", *Bristol Medico Chirurgical Journal* 1983, **98**, pp 104-108

2.   *Felix Farley's Bristol Journal* (strongly Tory) and *The Bristol Mercury* (Radical) both gave exactly the same report upon the 20th July 1833. Unlike the reporting of the cholera epidemics the reports of BMA meetings showed no political bias. The *Western Daily Press* (WDP) and *Mercury* carried similar reports of 1863 and '94, the latter, a weekly paper being shorter but similar in tone

3.   WDP, 5th August 1863

4.   A.J. Symonds. 1801-71, Physician to Bristol General Hospital. See biographical note by his son who edited a collection of his essays entitled *Miscellany*

5.   Augustin Prichard. Biographical details see below n.11

6.   Joseph Griffiths Swayne, Biographical details see below n.11. He chaired the section on obstetrics in 1894 and though the paper made some affectionate comments about him, it reported nothing on his subject

7.   William Budd, see note 12. Also E.W. Goodall, *William Budd*, Bristol 1936. E.E. Amory Wilson, *The Conquest of Epidemic Disease,* Princeton, 1943. D. Large & F. Round, *Public Health in Mid Victorian Bristol*, Bristol Branch of Historical Association, 1974. Margaret Pelling, *Cholera, Fever & English Medicine*, 1925-1865 Oxford, 1978

8.   Virus - Budd used this term as a general one for a transmissable, living, agent of disease.

9.   WDP, 8th August 1863, Symonds' home - Clifton Hill House

10. WDP, Tuesday 31st July 1894
     Institutions: 1. Bristol University College & Medical School 2. Bristol Royal Infirmary, 3 Bristol General Hospital 4. Bristol Childrens' Hospital 5. The Eye Hospital 6. Bristol Dispensary 7. Clifton Dispensary 8. Bristol Eye Dispensary 9. Bristol Medical Missionary Society 10. Bristol District Nurses' Society 11. West of England Sanatorium (Weston-super-Mare). These were of course all charities. No public, or mental hospitals are included

11. For biographical details see Geo. Munro Smith, *A History of the Bristol Royal Infirmary*, Bristol, 1917.

12. WDP, 1st August 1894, quoting Edward Long Fox's Presidential Address.

13. WDP, 4th August 1894: report of speech 3 columns; comment 1 column

14. WDP, (Editorial), 31st July 1894 - my italics

15. Social events were reported in some detail, the day after they took place

16. Thomas S Kuhn, *The Structure of Scientific Revolutions,* Chicago, 1962

ARTHUR CONAN DOYLE AND THE USE OF ENGLISH PROVINCIAL MEDICINE IN FICTION

Owen Dudley Edwards

The history of medicine very properly concerns itself with social history as well as intellectual history, or rather it recognises that these things are inextricably linked. And the social historian of any intellect should turn for instruction as well as for pleasure to examining fiction, an activity which was placed firmly on the historiographical agenda by the twenty-seven-year-old T. B. Macaulay in 1828 with particular reference to the value of the works of Sir Walter Scott.[1] Macaulay was here speaking of Scott as novelist of the past, but his own historical writing made good use of contemporary fictions among his sources, and these must be the chief area of interest. The historian of medicine is likely to derive more benefit from a close study of the lifestyle of Bob Sawyer, Ben Allen and their fellow-students of medicine in *The Pickwick Papers* than from a minute investigation of Dr Manette in *A Tale of Two Cities* in the hope of new insights on medicine in the *ancien regime*. Some historical novelists will always be of value for their insights and their researches into the past, notably Scott himself, or the elder Dumas, or Tolstoi. And whether writing of past or of present, some novelists of far poorer powers as novelists may have important evidence to produce which cannot be duplicated elsewhere. But both for enjoyment and for profit the historian of medicine is most fortunate in quarrying in the work of a master of fiction: a source which invites engagement with a mind worthy of respect stimulates the investigation in addition merely to feeding it.

Arthur Conan Doyle (1859-1930) is probably the finest of all such sources for the historian of British medicine. He was a successful general practitioner in Portsmouth from 1882 to 1890; he had graduated from the Edinburgh medical school as MB, BCh, in 1881, and as MD in 1885, thus having witnessed the last moments of its leadership over all other such institutions in the world. He was a professional writer who gave deep study to the traditions and techniques of the craft of fiction. Inevitably he drew on his medical knowledge: his Dr Watson is probably the most famous member of the medical fraternity in fiction, but his Sherlock Holmes is also the product of medical prototypes, several of them, although his own medical credentials are limited to extensive laboratory work, apparently in Bart's, and not a feature of any of the stories save the first, *A Study in Scarlet* (after which his laboratory experiments are chiefly conducted in 221B Baker Street). Conan Doyle's science-fiction novels and stories about Professor Challenger also draw heavily on the Edinburgh medical world of the 1870s, although the first of them, *The Lost World*, was not written until 1911.

The English provinces supplied him with a number of locations both for what he called his *Tales of Medical Life* and for stories, such as the Holmes cycle, in which he drew surreptitiously on his medical experience. Be it understood that "provinces" can only be the *English* provinces in such a situation: the concept is not a Scottish one, and as for the vulgar error which obtains so widely today in Government and media that Scotland is an

English province, to an Edinburgh medical man of the last century England as a whole was a Scottish province, in the Roman imperial sense of the term: an unenlightened place, with peculiar local superstitions and prejudices, needing to be nursed, judiciously evangelised, treated with a mixture of kindness and ferocity, and milked well. It could supply reputation and wealth, it might be judiciously flattered, but within the mind of its exploiter it must never be conceded scientific equality. Ostensibly, Conan Doyle did not write much about Scotland, although both in various reminiscences and in his haunting short story *The Captain of the Pole-Star* he drew ably and memorably on his student experience as medical attendant on a Scottish whaler in the waters of Greenland.[3]

Conan Doyle's experience of Portsmouth supplied his most obvious provincial location for his fiction, but both from personal knowledge and from extensive travelling and conversation he was able to draw on a much larger area. His ill-fated friendship with George Turnavine Budd introduced him not only to medical practice in Plymouth, but also to stories of the large family of doctors, Budd's father and uncles, who straddled Devonshire and adjoining locations as far afield as Bristol. They gave him some material for Dr James Mortimer of Dartmoor, in *The Hound of the Baskervilles*, as well as for other creations. He had brief experiences as a student assistant to doctors in Ruyton-in-Salop, and in Sheffield, and much more extensive residence in Birmingham in the same capacity. After residence in Norwood from 1891 to 1896 (broken by extensive travels in North America, Switzerland and Egypt), he moved to Hindhead, Surrey, and thence, in 1907, to Crowborough, Sussex. He knew north Lancashire well, from his days in the early 1870s as a schoolboy in Stonyhurst, and through his family's friendship with Dr Bryan Charles Waller, of Masongill, near Kirkby Lonsdale (who in Edinburgh days had first drawn him into medicine), Conan Doyle became well acquainted with the Yorkshire-Lancashire-Westmorland borders. He evidently drew out fellow-medics when he encountered them at public dinners or on other occasions, and thus could write with some authority on the provincial doctor in locations where his own experience was of the slightest: for instance *The Croxley Master*, a long story of a medical student driven to fight for a purse in a boxing tournament, is set in the Yorkshire collieries, to which his three weeks in Sheffield can only have supplied a nucleus.[4]

He was not always anxious to give too much assistance to the future historian in his scene-setting. When he drew on fact, some little disguise would be needed, and geographical transposition is a natural precaution. Many of his medical scenes are set in *Birchespool*, which certainly covers the identity of Portsmouth in his autobiographical novel *The Stark Munro Letters* (a work of value in its totality to students of Victorian provincial medicine and not discussed further here);[5] but other stories, all with different casts of characters, set in Birchespool, have features not present in Portsmouth. In *A Physiologist's Wife* it is a university town, which Portsmouth certainly was not.[6] The name, too, deriving from *Bir*mingham — Man*che*ster — Liver*pool*, is a warning that it is to be taken as a provincial city but not always as a specific one.

Locations are also deceptive in that some data are interchangeable with the London metropolis, and what is said of medicine in London, and even in Edinburgh, may sometimes hold good for the provinces. The omnipresent theme in Conan Doyle's fiction of the young, struggling professional whether in medicine or some other activity (including Sherlock Holmes's reminiscence of his first struggles as a consulting detective in *The Musgrave Ritual*) is often described with a London location but originates in its author's efforts to win a Portsmouth practice.[7] Conan Doyle's provinces, too, may be urban, small-town, village, or bleakly rural. But the key factor often lies in the relationship of provinces to metropolis. Sometimes a doctor may deliberately choose a provincial practice in preference to London, and Conan Doyle knew several who did. He may, like Dr James Ripley (*The Doctors of Hoyland*), have inherited a father's practice.[8] He may like Dr Mortimer of *The Hound of the Baskervilles* choose the provinces when marriage closes a hospital career to him and his own lack of ambition draws him to an agreeable and undemanding location. He may, like Dr Aloysius Lana (*The Black Doctor*), find a rural retreat a useful means to hide from an embarrassing family connection, or even, like Dr Cameron (*The Surgeon of Gaster Fell*), to hide the connection itself. But often the metropolis remains as the symbol of ambitions unfulfilled temporarily or permanently.

The most remarkable presentation of the provincial doctor, thirsting for recognition only the metropolis can normally bring, is found not in a medical guise but in the portrait of a detective. We must remember that not only Holmes but also the police detectives have their origin in Edinburgh doctors, and when Edinburgh had somewhat faded as an urgent influence, new detectives still showed antecedents in the profession their creator knew best. The provincial detective in the Holmes stories is in general no more ludicrous than the Scotland Yard variety (not that that says much for him), but Inspector Baynes in *Wisteria Lodge* is the only policeman who comes close to rivalling Holmes himself. He is no farther afield from London than rural Surrey but —

> Holmes smiled and rubbed his hands.
> "I must congratulate you, inspector, on handling so distinctive and instructive a case. Your powers, if I may say so without offence, seem superior to your opportunities."
> Inspector Baynes's small eyes twinkled with pleasure.
> "You're right, Mr Holmes. We stagnate in the provinces. A case of this sort gives a man a chance, and I hope that I shall take it. ..."

Baynes is also a conspicuous contrast to the usual police detectives in integrity. As a rule, apart from morons who refuse his assistance altogether, Holmes finds the police ready enough to accept his assistance on the understanding that they receive the credit: this is a convention of the stories from *A Study in Scarlet* to *The Retired Colourman* written forty years later. But not so Baynes:

> "You have a theory, then?"
> "And I'll work it myself, Mr Holmes. It's only due to my own credit to do so. Your name is made, but I have still to make mine. I should be glad to be able to say afterwards that I had solved it without your help."
> Holmes laughed good-humouredly.
> "Well, well, inspector", said he. "Do you follow your path and I will follow mine. My results are always very much at your service if you care to apply to me for them. ..."

Later Baynes releases a theory to the press which worries Holmes:

> "... Pray don't think it a liberty if I give you a word of friendly warning."
>
> "Of warning, Mr Holmes?"
>
> "I have looked into this case with some care, and I am not convinced that you are on the right lines. I don't want you to commit yourself too far, unless you are sure."
>
> "You're very kind, Mr Holmes."
>
> "I assure you I speak for your good."
>
> It seemed to me that something like a wink quivered for an instant over one of Mr Baynes's tiny eyes.
>
> "We agreed to work on our own lines, Mr Holmes. That's what I am doing."
>
> "Oh, very good", said Holmes. "Don't blame me."
>
> "No, sir; I believe you mean well by me. But we all have our own systems, Mr Holmes. You have yours, and maybe I have mine. ... You try yours and I will try mine. That's the agreement."
>
> Holmes shrugged his shoulders as we walked away together. "I can't make the man out. He seems to be riding for a fall. Well, as he says, we must each try our own way and see what comes of it. But there's something in Inspector Baynes which I can't quite understand."

Considering that Holmes himself had played the same trick of a bogus theory of the crime given to the press ("The Press, Watson, is a most valuable institution if you know how to use it."),[9] it might seem surprising that he would take Baynes, already marked down by him as possessed of fine powers, to have leaped to premature conclusions, but his lifelong experience of the official police clearly stood in the way of his concluding that Baynes was up to his own old games. Ultimately Baynes and Holmes prove to have arrived separately at the correct diagnosis.

> Holmes laid his hand upon the inspector's shoulder.
>
> "You will rise high in your profession. You have instinct and intuition", said he.
>
> Baynes flushed with pleasure.

It could be argued that Baynes's desire to prove himself the equal of Holmes was counter-productive in that for all of their accuracy and acumen, the villains ultimately escape them. Conan Doyle from time to time showed Holmes's enthusiasm for finding the correct solution leading to results of the case-was-a-success-but-the-patient-died variety,[10] or, as Conan Doyle himself phrased it in a medical story,[11]

> "Poor old Walker was very fond of experimental surgery, and he broke ground in several directions. Between ourselves, there may have been some more ground-breaking afterwards, but he did his best for his cases. ..."

Wisteria Lodge is not one of the best Holmes stories, being both unwieldy and, at times, illogical, but Conan Doyle seems to have been very anxious to pay this tribute to provincial intelligence and integrity.[12]

The metropolis in more formally medical contexts is also associated with claims of superiority against which the provinces are anxious where possible to assert themselves.

The Doctors of Hoyland is a remarkable vindication of the prowess of women doctors, and a shrewd discussion of their potential for success in conquest of a provincial practice, blending irony with romance with a fine pharmaceutical hand — the male chauvinist doctor who overcomes his prejudices finds his offer of marriage refused, firstly with the response "What, and unite the practices?", and then by the lady's gentle but firm insistence that:

> "... I intend to devote my life entirely to science. There are many women with a capacity for marriage, but few with a taste for biology. I will remain true to my own line, then. I came down here while waiting for an opening in the Paris Physiological Laboratory. I have just heard that there is a vacancy for me there, and so you will be troubled no more by my intrusion upon your practice. I have done you an injustice just as you did me one. I thought you narrow and pedantic, with no good quality. I have learned during your illness to appreciate you better, and the recollection of our friendship will always be a very pleasant one to me."

> And so it came about that in a very few weeks there was only one doctor in Hoyland. But folks noticed that the one had aged many years in a few months, that a weary sadness lurked always in the depths of his blue eyes, and that he was less concerned than ever with the eligible young ladies whom chance, or their careful country mammas, placed in his way.

When at an earlier point the injured Dr James Ripley is being attended by his female rival his brother hastens down from London:

> "... It struck me during the night that we may have been a little narrow in our views."
> "Nonsense, James. It's all very fine for women to win prizes in the lecture-room, but you know as well as I do that they are no use in an emergency. Now I warrant that this woman was all nerves when she was setting your leg. That reminds me that I had better just take a look at it and see that it is all right."
> "I would rather that you did not undo it", said the patient. "I have her assurance that it is all right".
> Brother William was deeply shocked.
> "Of course, if a woman's assurance is of more value than the opinion of the assistant surgeon of a London hospital, there is nothing more to be said", he remarked.
> "I should prefer that you did not touch it", said the patient firmly, and Doctor William went back to London that evening in a huff.

On the other hand Dr Hardacre, the country doctor in *The Brown Hand*, proves successful in his experiment by drawing on the resources of a London hospital where a friend is house-surgeon. As with Holmes and Baynes, the metropolis may offer useful assistance if integrity — or *amour-propre* — can permit of its acceptance. *The Doctors of Hoyland* is also an important reminder that the metropolis may be as bad as the provinces in clinging to discredited prejudices.[13]

The provincial doctor resembled his London colleague in private practice by owing much to the advantages of appearance.

Dr James Ripley was two-and-thirty years of age, reserved, learned, unmarried, and with set, rather stern features, and a thinning of the dark hair upon the top of his head, which was worth quite a hundred a year to him.

In London the fashionable doctor in attendance on the Foreign Secretary[14] is both more conscious of such advantages and better rewarded for their cultivation:[15]

He bowed in the courteous, sweeping, old-world fashion which had done so much to build up his ten thousand a year ...

He swung his golden *pince-nez* in his right hand as he walked, and bent forward with a peering, blinking expression, which was somehow suggestive of the dark and complex cases through which he had seen.

But the cultivation of appearance in the provinces was more closely in danger of covering hypocrisy, as revealed in the lethally etched portrait of Dr Oldacre (in *The Croxley Master*) who refuses a loan to his assistant to finance a return to college which would deprive Oldacre of his sweated labour:

He had prospered exceedingly by the support of the local Church interest, and the rule of his life was never by word or action to run a risk of offending the sentiment which had made him. His standard of respectability and of dignity was exceedingly high, and he expected the same from his assistants. ...
"You don't go to service, I observe, Mr Montgomery", said he coldly.
"No, sir; I have had some business to detain me."
"It is very near to my heart that my household should set a good example. There are so few educated people in this district that a great responsibility devolves upon us. If we do not live up to the highest, how can we expect these poor workers to do so?..."

But later:

"I should be glad if you could let me have leave for Saturday, Doctor Oldacre."
"It is very inconvenient upon so busy a day."
"I should do a double day's work on Friday so as to leave everything in order. I should hope to be back in the evening."
"I am afraid I cannot spare you, Mr Montgomery." ...
"You will remember, Doctor Oldacre, that when I came to you it was understood that I should have a clear day every month. I have never claimed one. But now there are reasons why I wish to have a holiday upon Saturday."
Doctor Oldacre gave in with a very bad grace.
"Of course, if you insist upon your formal rights, there is no more to be said, Mr Montgomery, though I feel that it shows a certain indifference to my comfort and the welfare of the practice. Do you still insist?"
"Yes, sir."
"Very good. Have your way."
The doctor was boiling over with anger, but Montgomery was a valuable assistant — steady, capable, and hard working — and he could not afford to lose him.

Oldacre's description of the practice, thus built up by sanctimonious professions and maintained by exploitation, is of one "intimately associated ... with the highest and most progressive elements of our small community", only to find it wounded both in pride and in pocket when Montgomery is discovered to have resorted to the boxing-ring:

> But just then the tentative bray of a cornet-player searching for his keynote jarred upon their ears, and an instant later the Wilson Colliery brass band was in full cry with *See the Conquering Hero Comes*, outside the surgery window. There was a banner waving, and a shouting crowd of miners.
> "What is it? What does it mean?" cried the angry doctor.
> "It means, sir, that I have, in the only way which was open to me, earned the money which is necessary for my education. It is my duty, Doctor Oldacre, to warn you that I am about to return to the University, and that you should lose no time in appointing my successor."

But it is clear Oldacre faces even greater dangers from his now lost assistant in the future, for after the victory Montgomery tells his backers when they try to persuade him to prolong his boxing career:

> "No; I have my own work to do now."
> "And what may that be?"
> "I'll use this money to get my medical degree."
> "Well, we've plenty of doctors, but you're the only man in the Riding that could smack the Croxley Master off his legs. However, I suppose you know your own business best. When you're a doctor, you'd best come down into these parts, and you'll always find a job waiting for you at the Wilson Coal-pits."

The sporting doctor had advantages not open to his more staid rivals, as Conan Doyle, a highly successful local cricketer, could testify. It is likely that he expected no such return when he looked for opportunities of relaxation in a manner long relished by him. But as a good observer he acknowledged its effects. Country doctors were less likely to assist themselves by prize-fighting, but on board ship he had found boxing a useful way of winning the respect of a tough crew, and registered it as a skill on which to draw if patients turned nasty.[16]

As a brilliant researcher Conan Doyle might be expected to make the case for the higher-qualified young struggling practitioner against the well-established but out-of-date seniors, and sometimes he did. The success of appearance against reality led him to produce the metaphor of a watch:

> That charming doctor, my dear madam, who pulled young Charley through the measles so nicely, and had such a pleasant manner and such a clever face, was a noted duffer at college and the laughing-stock of his year. While poor little Doctor Grinder whom you snubbed so, and who seemed so nervous and didn't know where to put his hands, he won a gold medal for original research and was as good a man as his professors. After all, it is generally the outside case, not the inside works, which is noticed in this world.

And in the same story, *Crabbe's Practice*, Crabbe, a thinly-disguised George Budd, complains:

> "... I wouldn't mind if these other fellows were good men, but they are not. They are all antiquated old fogies at least half a century behind the day. Now there is old Markham, who lives in that brick house over there and does most of the practice in the town. I'll swear he doesn't know the difference between locomotor ataxia and a hypodermic syringe, but he is known, so they flock to his surgery in a manner which is simply repulsive. And Davidson down the road, he is only an LSA. Talked about epispastic paralysis at the Society the other night — confused it with liquor epispasticus, you know. Yet that fellow makes a pound to my shilling."

That was written in 1884. But ten years later he did not include it in his book of medical tales, *Round the Red Lamp*,[17] for which he had written *Behind the Times* telling a very different lesson. It concludes, after giving a sketch of the elderly, reactionary Dr Winter whom the narrator has literally known from his own birth:

> When Dr Patterson and I, both of us young, energetic, and up-to-date, settled in the district, we were most cordially received by the old doctor, who would have been only too happy to be relieved of some of his patients. The patients themselves, however, followed their own inclinations, which is a reprehensible way that patients have, so that we remained neglected with our modern instruments and our latest alkaloids, while he was serving out senna and calomel to all the countryside. We both of us loved the old fellow, but at the same time, in the privacy of our own intimate conversations, we could not help commenting upon this deplorable lack of judgment.
>
> "It is all very well for the poorer people", said Patterson, "but after all the educated classes have a right to expect that their medical man will know the difference between a mitral murmur and a bronchitic râle. It's the judicial frame of mind, not the sympathetic, which is the essential one."
>
> I thoroughly agreed with Patterson in what he said. It happened, however, that very shortly afterwards the epidemic of influenza broke out, and we were all worked to death. One morning I met Patterson on my round, and found him looking rather pale and fagged out. He made the same remark about me. I was in fact feeling far from well, and I lay upon the sofa all afternoon with a splitting headache and pains in every joint. As evening closed in I could no longer disguise the fact that the scourge was upon me, and I felt that I should have medical advice without delay. It was of Patterson naturally that I thought, but somehow the idea of him had suddenly become repugnant to me. I thought of his cold, critical attitude, of his endless questions, of his tests and his tappings. I wanted something more soothing — something more genial.
>
> "Mrs Hudson", said I to my housekeeper, "would you kindly run along to old Dr Winter and tell him that I should be obliged to him if he would step round."
>
> She was back with an answer presently.
>
> "Dr Winter will come round in an hour or so, sir, but he has just been called in to attend Dr Patterson."

To a patient — perhaps not to a doctor — it is hard to read those lines without some slight constriction of the throat and a little watering of the eyes. As George Bernard Shaw pointed out in his dramatic criticism of the play *Waterloo* based by Conan Doyle on his short story *A Straggler of '15*, Conan Doyle was a master of pathos within comedy.[18] Reprinted in his *Tales of Adventure and Medical Life* (1922) it would naturally have attracted the attention of writers studying the established traditions of medical fiction, and seems the most likely origin of the soap-opera convention of impetuous, modern, young doctor and canny, experienced, old doctor - as in the Scottish TV series (based on A.J. Cronin's novels) *Dr Finlay's Casebook*, the US's *Ben Casey* and *Dr Kildare*, U S radio's *Young Dr Malone*, and the movies based on Richard Gordon's *Doctor* series. The convention in fact became so strong that Sir Lancelot Spratt who first lived and died in Gordon's *Doctor in the House* with virtually no resemblance to Dr Winter was resurrected in later novels to play a part redrawn in somewhat Winter contours first inhabited by James Robertson Justice's creation of the part on screen. There is less dignity to the Spratt metamorphosis than to Conan Doyle's Dr Winter, but after all the original Spratt is introduced in a Maupassant-like episode: Dr Cameron in *Finlay* and Dr Gillespie in *Kildare*, while less archaic than Dr Winter, are obvious relatives. Consider:

> He had been trained also at a time when instruments were in a rudimentary state and when men learned to trust more to their own fingers. He has a model surgical hand, muscular in the palm, tapering in the fingers, "with an eye at the end of each". I shall not easily forget how Dr Patterson and I cut Sir John Sirwell, the County Member,[19] and were unable to find the stone. It was a horrible moment. Both our careers were at stake. And then it was that Dr Winter, whom we had asked out of courtesy to be present, introduced into the wound a finger which seemed to our excited senses to be about nine inches long, and hooked out the stone at the end of it.
> "It's always well to bring one in your waistcoat pocket", said he with a chuckle, "but I suppose you youngsters are above all that."

The Sherlockologist will of course light enthusiastically on the name of the narrator's housekeeper, Mrs Hudson, famous in Conan Doyle fiction as that of Holmes and Watson's landlady. It is highly suggestive that in rapidly reaching for a suitable name for a housekeeper while high-lighting the tension of the modern scientific method in opposition to the old-fashioned humanitarian, Conan Doyle's mind glided into 221B Baker Street. For the Holmes-Watson partnership in part is based on the same tension as revealed, for instance, thus:[20]

> I could not but observe that, as she took the seat which Sherlock Holmes placed for her, her lip trembled, her hand quivered, and she showed every sign of intense inward agitation. ...
> "... from that day to this no word has ever been heard of my unfortunate father. He came home, with his heart full of hope, to find some peace, some comfort, and instead ..." She put her hand to her throat, and a choking sob cut short the sentence.
> "The date?" asked Holmes, opening his note-book.

The Holmes stories are greatly misunderstood if it is not realised that Watson's humane decency is intended to give the reader identification with him through first-person narrative thus getting some perspective despite the remoteness of Holmes. We actually have means of seeing Watson's methods of research in *The Hound of the Baskervilles* in which he makes excellent observations of emotional phenomena, Mrs Barrymore's grief in the night as revealed by her swollen eyelids, Mrs Laura Lyons's expectation of a visitor to whom she was attracted and the underlying sensuality of her facial expression. Scientific analysis of human beings undertaken without human sympathy is something which Conan Doyle seemed to feel peculiarly inapplicable to the provinces where a sense of common humanity was needed in medical watch over the community. He satirised the former in *A False Start*:[21]

> Whilst the doctor had been running his eyes over the stranger, the latter had been plunging his hands into pocket after pocket of his heavy coat. The heat of the weather, his dress, and this exercise of pocket rummaging had all combined to still further redden his face, which had changed from brick to beet, with a gloss of moisture on his brow. This extreme ruddiness brought a clue at last to the observant doctor. Surely it was not to be attained without alcohol. In alcohol lay the secret of this man's trouble. Some little delicacy was needed, however, in showing him that he had read his case aright, that at a glance he had penetrated to the inmost sources of his ailments.
> "It's very hot", observed the stranger, mopping his forehead.
> "Yes. It is weather which tempts one to drink rather more beer than is good for one", answered Doctor Horace Wilkinson looking very knowingly at his companion from over his finger-tips.
> "Dear! dear! You shouldn't do that."
> "I! I never touch beer."
> "Neither do I. I've been an abstainer for twenty years."
> This was depressing. Doctor Wilkinson blushed until he was nearly as red as the other.

If the Sherlock Holmes stories celebrated the genius of Conan Doyle's Edinburgh teacher, Joseph Bell, in somewhat flamboyantly deducing all manner of data of medical relevance and irrelevance from patients' appearance, *A False Start* questions the value of such proceedings. On the other hand, old Dr Winter's methods succeed despite their archaism because of their concern with the remedial value of the doctor's contrivances to soothe the patient, not their use for showy demonstrations of cleverness or artistic revelations of profundity:

> ... at last there came a time of real illness — a time when I lay for months together inside my wicker-work basket bed, and then it was that I learned that that hard face could relax, that those country-made, creaking boots could steal very gently to a bedside, and that that rough voice could thin into a whisper when it spoke to a sick child.

> ... His mere presence leaves the patient with more hopefulness and vitality. The sight of disease affects him as dust does a careful housewife. It makes him angry and impatient. "Tut, tut, this will never do!" he cries, as he takes over a new case. He would shoo death out of the room as though he were an intrusive hen. But when

the intruder refuses to be dislodged, when the blood moves more slowly and the eyes grow dimmer, then it is that Dr Winter is of more avail than all the drugs in his surgery. Dying folk cling to his hand as if the presence of his bulk and vigour gives them more courage to face the change; and that kindly, wind-beaten face has been the last earthly impression that many a sufferer has carried into the unknown.

On one of Dr Winter's attainments Conan Doyle singled out a phenomenon which patients know, if they are lucky, wherever they live:

> He has the healing touch — that magnetic thing which defies explanation or analysis, but which is a very evident fact none the less.

(*Experto crede*: how did my own family doctor, the late George Buchanan of Dublin, give me innumerable injections when I was a child with infinitely less pain than those administered by any other doctor, save his daughter Joan who ultimately inherited his practice?)

The doctor in the Victorian provinces, in the observation of the former Catholic Conan Doyle, became something like the secular priest of his or her community. The more limited range of distractions, pleasures, strata of society, all drew the community closer together, increased their dependence on one another, and immunised them against centrifugal forces. The secular priest could be as hollow in his vocation as Dr Oldacre, or as dependent on dubious trickery as certain other Conan Doyle characters, but the principle remained. Several stories in which a doctor makes a fleeting appearance make it clear that a wise and loving mother, wife or relative often made far more difference to a patient's comfort and survival than any doctor, and that such women were often shrewd analysts of the proportions of wheat and chaff to be harvested from a doctor's visit. Hence in his description of a woman doctor he singled out the very qualities by which women in the home had for so long and with so little thanks done so much of the doctor's work: common sense, nerve, delicacy, gentleness.

> Farmer Eyton, whose callous ulcer had been quietly spreading over his shin for years back under a gentle *régime* of zinc ointment, was painted round with blistering fluid, and found, after three blasphemous nights, that his sore was stimulated into healing. Mrs Crowder, who had always regarded the birth-mark upon her second daughter Eliza as a sign of the indignation of the Creator at a third helping of raspberry tart which she had partaken of during a critical period, learned that, with the help of two galvanic needles, the mischief was not irreparable. ... what galled [Dr Ripley] most of all was, when she did something which he had pronounced to be impracticable. For all his knowledge, he lacked nerve as an operator, and usually sent his worst cases up to London. The lady, however, had no weakness of this sort, and took everything that came in her way. It was agony to him to hear that she was about to straighten little Alec Turner's club foot, and right at the fringe of the rumour came a note from his mother, the rector's wife, asking him if he would be so good as to act as chloroformist. It would be inhumanity to refuse, as there was no other who could take the place, but it was gall and wormwood to his sensitive nature. Yet, in spite of his vexation, he could not but

admire the dexterity with which the thing was done. She handled the little wax-foot so gently, and held the tiny tenotomy knife as an artist holds his pencil. One straight insertion, one snick of a tendon, and it was all over without a stain upon the white towel which lay beneath.

The woman doctor, Dr Verrinder Smith, succeeds in part because of her deployment of the latest science against provincial superstition. Dr Winter, whom in some respects she resembles, succeeds in spite of fifty years' progress. Yet in his case the history of medicine is justified for the most practical purposes because of the antiquity of his experience and its survival as more than a walking museum.

Fifty years have brought him little and deprived him of less. Vaccination was well within the teaching of his youth, though I think he has a secret preference for inoculation. Bleeding he would practice freely but for public opinion. Chloroform he regards as a dangerous innovation, and he always clicks with his tongue when it is mentioned. He has even been known to say vain things about Laennec, and to refer to the stethoscope as "a newfangled French toy". He carries one in his hat out of deference to the expectations of his patients; but he is very hard of hearing, so that it makes little difference whether he uses it or not. ...

He is so very much behind the day that occasionally, as things move round in their usual circle, he finds himself, to his own bewilderment, in the front of the fashion. Dietetic treatment, for example, had been much in vogue in his youth, and he has more practical knowledge of it than anyone whom I have met. Massage, too, was familiar to him when it was new to our generation.

These last points are most useful charts for the historian, as well as indications that remedies lost to fashion or roads of medical progress by-passed in former days may well justify their rediscovery.

The fiction of Conan Doyle offers lessons charged by his idealism:[22]

"... a doctor has very much to be thankful for also. Don't you ever forget it. It is such a pleasure to do a little good that a man should pay for the privilege instead of being paid for it. Still, of course, he has his home to keep up and his wife and children to support. But his patients are his friends — or they should be so. He goes from house to house, and his step and his voice are loved and welcomed in each. What could a man ask for more than that? And besides, he is forced to be a good man. It is impossible for him to be anything else. How can a man spend his whole life in seeing suffering bravely borne and yet remain a hard or a vicious man? It is a noble, generous, kindly profession, and you youngsters have got to see that it remains so."

But it also knew what the provinces could contain:[23]

Holmes had been buried in the morning papers all the way down, but after we had passed the Hampshire border he threw them down, and began to admire the scenery. It was an ideal spring day, a light blue sky, flecked with little fleecy white clouds drifting across from west to east. The sun was shining very brightly, and yet there was an exhilarating nip in the air, which set an edge to a man's energy. All over the countryside, away to the rolling hills around Aldershot, the little red and grey roofs of the farm-steadings peeped out from amidst the light green of the new foliage.

"Are they not fresh and beautiful?" I cried, with all the enthusiasm of a man fresh from the fogs of Baker Street.

But Holmes shook his head gravely.

"Do you know, Watson", said he, "that it is one of the curses of a mind with a turn like mine that I must look at everything with reference to my own special subject. You look at these scattered houses, and you are impressed by their beauty. I look at them, and the only thought which comes to me is a feeling of their isolation, and of the impunity with which crime may be committed there."

"Good heavens!" I cried. "Who would associate crime with these dear old homesteads?"

"They always fill me with a certain horror. It is my belief, Watson, founded upon my experience, that the lowest and vilest alleys in London do not present a more dreadful record of sin than does the smiling and beautiful countryside."

"You horrify me!"

"But the reason is very obvious. The pressure of public opinion can do in the town what the law cannot accomplish. There is no lane so vile that the scream of a tortured child, or the thud of a drunkard's blow, does not beget sympathy and indignation among the neighbours, and then the whole machinery of justice is ever so close that a word of complaint can set it going, and there is but a step between the crime and the dock. But look at these lonely houses, each in its own fields, filled for the most part with poor ignorant folk who know little of the law. Think of the deeds of hellish cruelty, the hidden wickedness which may go on, year in, year out, in such places, and none the wiser. ..."

BIBLIOGRAPHY

Listed in the following order:-

Publication Date	Title	Magazine	Month	First Book Publication	Omnibus Vol.
1883	*The Captain of the Pole-Star*	Temple Bar	January	The Captain of the Pole Star (1890)	The Conan Doyle Stories
1884	*Crabbe's Practice*	Boy's Own Paper	Christmas	Tales of Adventure and Medical Life (1922)	The Conan Doyle Stories
1887	*A Study in Scarlet*	Beeton's Christmas Annual		A Study in Scarlet (1888)	Complete Sherlock Holmes
1890	*The Sign of the Four*	Lippincott's	February	The Sign of Four (1890)	Complete Sherlock Holmes
1890	*A Physiologist's Wife*	Blackwood's	September	Round the Red Lamp (1894)	The Conan Doyle Stories
1890	*The Surgeon of Gaster Fell*	Chambers' Journal	December	Danger! (1918) (shorthand)	The Conan Doyle Stories
1891	*A Straggler of '15*	Black and Whites	March	Round the Red Lamp (1894)	The Conan Doyle Stories
1891	*A False Start*	Gentlewoman	Christmas	Round the Red Lamp (1894)	none
1892	*The Copper Beeches*	Strand	June	The Adventures of Sherlock Holmes (1892)	Complete Sherlock Holmes
1892	*A Question of Diplomacy*	Illustrated London News	Summer	Round the Red Lamp (1894)	none
1893	*The Musgrave Ritual*	Strand	May	The Memoirs of Sherlock Holmes (1893)	Complete Sherlock Holmes
1894	*The Doctors of Hoyland*	Idler	April	Round the Red Lamp (1894)	The Conan Doyle Stories
1894	*Behind the Times*	none	none	Round the Red Lamp (1894)	The Conan Doyle Stories
1894	*The Surgeon Talks*	none	none	Round the Red Lamp (1894)	The Conan Doyle Stories
1894-95	*The Stark Munro Letters*	Idler	October-November	The Stark Munro Letters (1895)	none
1898	*The Beetle Hunter*	Strand	June	Round the Fire Stories (1908)	The Conan Doyle Stories
1898	*The Black Doctor*	Strand	October	Round the Fire Stories (1908)	The Conan Doyle Stories
1899	*The Brown Hand*	Strand	May	Round the Fire Stories (1908)	The Conan Doyle Stories
1899	*The Croxley Master*	Strand	October-December	The Green Flag (1900)	The Conan Doyle Stories
1901-02	*The Hound of the Baskervilles*	Strand	August-April	The Hound of the Baskervilles (1902)	Complete Sherlock Holomes
1904	*The Six Napoleons*	Strand	May	The Return of Sherlock Holmes	Complete Sherlock Holmes
1907	*Waterloo* (play)	none	none	Waterloo (1907)	none
1908	*Wisteria Lodge*	Strand	September-October	His Last Bow (1917)	Complete Sherlock Holmes
1912	*The Lost World*	Strand	April-October	The Lost World (1912)	Complete Professor Challenger
1927	*The Retired Colourman*	Strand	January	The Case-Book of Sherlock Holmes (1927)	Complete Sherlock Holmes

NOTES AND REFERENCES

1.   "History", *Edinburgh Review* (May 1828), 331-67. The Essay is not included by him in his *Critical and Historical Essays* but may be found in the posthumous *Miscellaneous Writings* ed T F Ellis (1860): a useful abridgement of it may be studied in the context of other historians' philosophies in Fritz Stern ed, *The Varieties of History from Voltaire to the Present* (1956), 71-89. Arthur Conan Doyle, *Through the Magic Door* (1907), 10-46, contains some very perceptive appreciation of Macaulay and Scott, and is a most instructive example of a professional writer's reflections on his reading.

2.   I have discussed the influence of Conan Doyle's youth in Edinburgh and Stonyhurst on his writings in my *The Quest for Sherlock Holmes - a Biographical Study of Sir Arthur Conan Doyle* (1983). The invaluable Richard Lancelyn Green and John Michael Gibson, *A Bibliography of A Conan Doyle* (1983) is a pleasure to use: I have extracted from it the chronological list of Conan Doyle's writings mentioned in the text. See also R Lancelyn Green ed, *The Uncollected Sherlock Holmes* (1983). Geoffrey Stavert, *A Study in Southsea - The Unrevealed Life of Doctor Arthur Conan Doyle* (1987), chronicles Conan Doyle's career in the Southsea district of Portsmouth, and Alvin E Rodin and Jack D Key, *Medical Casebook of Doctor Arthur Conan Doyle* (1984), is a deeply researched study of the medical content of his life and writings, although neither is as reliable as the *Bibliography*.

3.   Details of publication of Conan Doyle's fictional writings cited here are given in the chronological guide included with this article. On Greenland see my chapter 8, "The Long Voyage Home", *Quest for Sherlock Holmes*, and Conan Doyle, "Life on a Greenland Whaler", *Strand* (January 1897), reprinted with some alterations as chapter 4 of his *Memories and Adventures* (1924, 1930). "Black Peter" in *The Return of Sherlock Holmes* makes some use of whaling. For his Scottish stories, see chiefly my brief collection *The Edinburgh Stories of Arthur Conan Doyle* (1981), "The Man from Archangel" (available in The Conan Doyle Stories) and "Our Midnight Visitor" (in *The Unknown Conan Doyle: Uncollected Stories* edd J M Gibson and R Lancelyn Green). Rodin and Key, *Medical Casebook*, is far-reaching and comprehensive in calendaring the whole range of medical allusions in Conan Doyle's fiction: as they point out medicine is sometimes of little importance to his plots when the chief protagonist is a medical student or doctor (eg in "Our Midnight Visitor").

4.   I examine the Stonyhurst, Waller and Budd connections in my *Quest for Sherlock Holmes*.

5.   *The Stark Munro Letters* is so firmly based on autobiography (not, admittedly, to the extent of the infallibility on every detail and conversation with which Hesketh Pearson credits it in his *Conan Doyle* (1943)) that it raises different questions from those of straightforward fiction: some incidents in the formal fictions are clearly autobiographical but their setting outside of their author's life gives greater freedom to their use. The book should be read in conjunction with *Memories and*

Adventures, chapters 6 to 9. On Conan Doyle's capacity for transposition of location the most obvious case is *A Study in Scarlet* where much Edinburgh material is presented as of London (see my *Quest for Sherlock Holmes* and my *Dr Jekyll and Mr Holmes*).

6. "A Physiologist's Wife", written in 1885, is another example of transposition, being fairly obviously derived from reflection on Edinburgh academic life: Conan Doyle pointed out (*Memories and Adventures*, p 88) that it "was written when I was under the influence of Henry James", a polite way of saying that it is in part gently satirical at James's expense, its very ambiguous heroine being "Mrs O'James".

7. To take only the Sherlock Holmes stories, the failed, struggling or near-impoverished professional may be found in the first two collections thus: pawnbroker (*The Red-Headed League*), journalist (*The Man with the Twisted Lip*), literary hack (*The Blue Carbuncle*), engineer (*The Engineer's Thumb*), governess (*The Copper Beeches*), stockbroker (*The Stockbroker's Clerk*), banker (*The Gloria Scott*), detective and schoolmaster (*The Musgrave Ritual*), doctor (*The Resident Patient*), diplomat (*The Naval Treaty*), and, of course, professor (*The Final Problem*): twelve examples from 24 stories.

8. Inheritance of a father's practice is anything but a sinecure in the fiction of Conan Doyle. In *The Doctors of Hoyland* Dr Ripley nearly loses his inheritance to his female rival and is saved only by her departure. Nor is there security in the inheritance of a great medical name in the locality. Bishop's Crossing in *The Black Doctor* is ten miles from Liverpool: "The practice of that district had been in the hands of Edward Rowe, the son of Sir William Rowe, the Liverpool consultant, but he had not inherited the talents of his father, and Dr Lana, with his advantages of presence and of manner, soon beat him out of the field." Conan Doyle's experience of Budd's struggles had shown how little use a great name in the previous generation might be. It gave some advantages when the inheritor capitalised on them, thus of Dr Ripley's initial rivals "one had sickened and wasted, being, as it was said, himself the only patient whom he had treated during his eighteen months of ruralising. A second had bought a fourth share of a Basingstoke practice, and had departed honourably, while a third had vanished one September night, leaving a gutted house and an unpaid drug bill behind him."

9. "The Six Napoleons" (*The Return of Sherlock Holmes*).

10. *Quest for Sherlock Holmes*, p 200.

11. *The Surgeon Talks*. The surgeon, Smith, whose monologue supplies the entire text, is London-based but like all of Conan Doyle's London medical material it may be searched with profit for content of Edinburgh and English provincial relevance.

12. I have used the *Strand* texts throughout in quoting from the Sherlock Holmes stories, otherwise I use first book publication. *Wisteria Lodge* was written after two years (1906 - 1908) in which Conan Doyle's first wife died, he remarried, he travelled extensively and moved from Surrey to Sussex, and he wrote very little

fiction. (*Holmes's Return* followed a decade (1894 - 1903) of almost incessant fictional writing.)   Some of its weaknesses are indicated in D Martin Dakin, *A Sherlock Holmes Commentary* (1972), pp 218-20, and they impair suspension of disbelief as seldom happens elsewhere in the cycle. Apart from Baynes, *Wisteria Lodge* is chiefly distinguished by its presentation of an English worthy as an obvious advantage around which to build an alibi, and Miss Burnet's "What does the law of England care for the rivers of blood shed years ago in San Pedro ...? To you they are like crimes committed in some other planet." Conan Doyle was on the eve of embroilment in agitation against the crimes and forced labour in King Leopold's Congo.

13. Conan Doyle did not go in much for the Dickensian-Trollopeian use of self-descriptive surnames, but "Hardacre" is a nice touch for an "impecunious" country doctor.

14. Styled "The Foreign Minister", a precaution also observed in the Holmes story *The Naval Treaty*.

15. *A Question of Diplomacy*.

16. Stavert, *A Study in Southsea*, is a fund of information on Conan Doyle's sporting career as a provincial doctor.   There is a nice piece of symbolism in *The Croxley Master* which catches the yearning of the struggling provincial doctor (not only the impoverished medical student of the story) to confront a human obstacle, however formidable, in place of the amorphous barriers to his professional success:

> Any nervousness which he may have had completely passed away now that he had his work before him. Here was something definite — this hard-faced, deformed Hercules to beat, with a career as the price of beating him. He glowed with the joy of action; it thrilled through his nerves.

17. *Crabbe's Practice* is unique in Conan Doyle's writing in having to wait almost forty years for book publication, which it received in *Tales of Adventure and Medical Life*, the relevant volume of a collected edition of short stories neither about Holmes nor (save two) about Brigadier Gerard: all volumes were later included in the omnibus *The Conan Doyle Stories*. It celebrates Budd, and so may have been really obnoxious to Conan Doyle's mother who detested Budd and died the year before its book publication: the treatment of Budd (as Cullingworth) in *The Stark Munroe Letters* is justly severe. Conan Doyle may have omitted it from the obvious place, *Round the Red Lamp* partly because of Crabbe's opportunism which so strikingly conflicts with the idealism of the volume which, as it stands, does not weaken its realism, humour and irony. He was also about to bring out *The Stark Munro Letters* in the *Idler* where many of the stories of *Round the Red Lamp* first appeared, and may not have wished to exhibit two characters, Crabbe and Cullingworth, so clearly from one source. Several stories in *Round the Red Lamp* proved too grim for inclusion in the *Idler*, being, said Conan Doyle "strictly — some would say too strictly — realistic": *His First Operation*, *The Third Generation* (on inherited consequences of syphilis), *The Curse of Eve* (on childbirth), *A*

Medical Document (reminiscences of three doctors) and *The Surgeon Talks* (reminiscence by one). Lancelyn Green and Gibson comment (*Bibliography*, p 82): "Even so he had toned down the more melodramatic moments. In the original version of "The Curse of Eve", which he read at the Authors' Club, the wife died leaving her husband accusing the newly born child of murder. In the revised form the wife recovered." He still retained something of the feeling:

"Kiss it, Robert!" cried the grandmother. "Kiss your son!"
But he felt a resentment to the little, red, blinking creature. He could not forgive it yet for that long night of misery. He caught sight of a white face in the bed and he ran towards it with such love and pity as his speech could find no words for.

18.   Shaw, "Mr Irving Takes Paregoric", *Saturday Review* 11 May 1895 (*Bibliography*, pp 148-49). Henry Irving had received great applause for his performance of the nonagenarian Waterloo veteran but Shaw stated: "The entire effect is contrived by the author, and it is due to him alone." The story has a nice medical cameo:

The doctor smiled.
"Well, you are doing very well", said he. "I'll look in once a week or so and see how you are!" As Norah followed him to the door he beckoned her outside. "He is very weak", he whispered. "If you find him failing you must send for me."
"What ails him, doctor?"
"Ninety years ail him. His arteries are pipes of lime. His heart is shrunken and flabby. The man is worn out."

19.   One must always be alive to Conan Doyle's sparkling but not necessarily obtrusive sense of fun. The obvious origin of this line is the old phrase much used in Victorian melodramatic fiction whereby a social outcast is "cut by the County". The struggling provincial doctor must often have felt himself to be in the same situation as the social outcast.

20.   *The Sign of Four*, chapter 2.

21.   A variant of the misreading of tell-tale signs is given in *Stark Munro*, chapter 13, which indicates an autobiographical origin, but not including this particular diagnosis. Conan Doyle from his father's tragedy knew all too much about signs of alcoholism to be mistaken in reading them. (*Quest for Sherlock Holmes*, pp 209-10).

22.   These are the closing lines of *The Surgeon Talks* and with them closes *Round the Red Lamp*. The positioning is clearly intentional.

23.   *The Copper Beeches*.

Index